The Complete Teething Guide

78/100

From Birth to Adolescence

*Offering Parents Healthy Alternatives
for Teething-Related Symptoms*

By
Kathy Arnos

Foreword by
Jay Gordon, M.D.

愛

Spirit Dance Publishing
Van Nuys, California

Library of Congress Control Number
2003095365
The complete teething guide: from birth to adolescence/ by Kathy Arnos, foreword by
Jay Gordon, M.D., tooth fairy illustrations by Nicole Pisaniello; photographs by Kathy
Arnos, Danielle Arnos, Mary Fuentes and Darick Nordstrom, D.D.S.;
charts and diagrams by Kathy Arnos – First edition.
Includes bibliographical references and index.

ISBN 09725783-6-6

Spirit Dance Publishing,
P.O. Box 1029-198, Van Nuys, CA 91408.
www.spiritdancepublishing.com
www.teething.us

First printing September 2003
Published in the United States of America

I would like to dedicate this book to the
children of the world who have been
misunderstood or mislabeled by our society.
This book is for you!

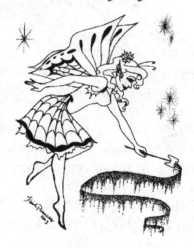

In loving memory of my parents,
Rose and Dan Barmish.

Disclaimer

This book contains advice and information relating to diet, nutrition, homeopathic and flower essence remedies for children and women. Although the homeopathic and flower remedies offered in this book are considered safe, it is impossible to predict any one child or adult's individual response to their use. This book is not intended to take the place of seeking professional medical attention when necessary. It should only be used as a reference in an ongoing partnership between doctor, dentist and patient (or patient's parent). The author and publisher disclaim all responsibility for any effects that may occur as a result of advice in context to this book. You should contact a qualified health care professional for any medical questions or emergencies.

Acknowledgements

The truth is no one ever writes a book alone. It is a collective effort that is the result of a vision, passion, observation or experience that needs to be expressed and shared with others. So when a different idea comes along and needs nurturing, it usually takes an eclectic crowd to bring the pieces of the puzzle together. I have been very fortunate in having an amazing group of angels on my team. I would like to thank Spirit for divinely guiding each of those special people to my table with their symptoms, stories, expertise, wisdom, patience, honesty and the courage to open their minds.

My deepest gratitude goes to my daughter Danielle, who continues to teach me daily, from her early years through young womanhood. I thank you for putting up with taking one more homeopathic remedy in the face of adversity. Your physical symptoms and emotional behavior in relation to the teething process have been my most precious learning experience. It was only though our personal journey, that I was able to help other parents address their children's health and emotional issues.

I want to extend a special thank you to an angel who has been with me since I began my writing career: Laura Barnaby, your devotion to our friendship is a blessing. There are no words for my appreciation of your amazing editing skills and for being the best midwife I could have asked for in birthing this book. Thanks also to: My dear friend Lynne Walker, R.Ph., for your insights and for being a messenger over the years; Jacqui Nimitz for getting me organized in the transition phase; David Howard for your skillful graphic work, Erin Gray for the *woo* way and standing waves that keep me grounded and centered; Dave Bower for always being the voice of reason and knowing that a lavender rose smells like the color purple – you are my Spirit dance; Kim Basinger for your enthusiasm and support in all my work; and all the practitioners and friends who were just a phone call away, Christine Vaughn, D.C., Parissa Ezzati, D.D.S., (and staff), Jay Gordon, M.D., Paul Fleiss, M.D., Charles Greenwood, D.C., Raven Montijo, L.Ac, Donna Yerman, D.C., (thanks for packing the parachute), Debbie Cholodenko, D.C., Mark Harmon, D.D.S., Kenneth

Stoller, M.D., Rowan Richards, D.C., Michael Harris, Mac Guru, Anh at the Photoshop, Nichie, and TipTop printing staff, as well as all the other practitioners not mentioned who contributed their expertise and wisdom. I also want to thank the authors who have written before me that have helped provide the knowledge within these pages. And last, but certainly not least, all my clients who have shared their stories and helped me learn a clearer truth about our children. For all of you, I am grateful!

Contents

A Healthy Start: Building a Solid Foundation
Nutrition During Pregnancy
Tooth Structure
Basic Nutrition Components
Nutrition for The Newborn – Adolescence

A Teething Timeline
A Traditional View – Natal and Neonatal Teeth
Understanding Emotional, Spiritual & Physical Growth Patterns
Timeline Chart

Breastfeeding - Bottle-feeding
How They Affect Tooth and Jaw Development
Physiological Differences
Nutritional Differences
Infant Formula
Bottle Mouth Syndrome
Thumb Sucking
Pacifiers

Foreword

"It's just teething." I said these words many times to new parents during my early years as a pediatrician when they were calling me or visiting my office to tell me that their babies were very uncomfortable, cranky, sleeping or eating less, biting, or ... all of these!

I will never use that phrase again lightly because it diminishes the importance and impact of teething, which is one of the most important phases in the first years of life. The phrase 'just teething' simply underestimates crucial anatomical and physiological changes that begin in infancy and continue into the teenage and young adult years.

As I read *The Complete Teething Guide*, I found myself learning much more in a few short hours than I had gleaned from several years of pediatric training and practice. This book gave me a valuable refresher course on the nutritional aspects of teething and tooth formation and a solid chronology of the way baby teeth come in, and how they are replaced, renewed and replenished.

Perhaps the most important information centers on how to deal with the "middle-of-the-night" issues, showing parents how they can help babies and children with teething pain, teething mood swings and even illness. I agree with Kathy that the stress of teething can and does affect the way the immune system fights off childhood illnesses. Both standard and alternative remedies are evaluated and discussed. *The Complete Teething Guide* provides good reading and good information for doctors and patients alike. (I hope your doctor reads this book, but I'm not optimistic: Summarize the key points and tell him or her about them!)

Other important issues addressed include fluoride and orthodontics. I don't think babies and children should receive fluoride supplements and my ambivalence about dental sealants was confirmed by research shared within these pages. Also, in my practice, I get daily questions about orthodontia and Kathy answers these questions better than I ever could.

This very readable book has a wealth of practical advice, whether it's choosing a dentist or a toothbrush and toothpaste and makes sure that these common questions are addressed thoroughly and intelligently. The section on hazards and emergency matters is very well done and, again, helped me remember the key points I'd learned in my training.

Equally important to me, though, is an emphasis of breastfeeding's beneficial effect on dental health and cavity prevention. There are still doctors and dentists who don't know that breast milk nourishes teeth and, instead, tell mothers they must stop nursing at night or their babies will get more cavities. This book may a go a long way towards educating parents and their doctors and might even reverse this illogical and scientific attitude. Would Mother Nature actually have made the mistake of making mother's milk a carcinogenic (decay-causing) food? Or course not.

Kathy's book answers questions parents ask me every day. Now I have better answers for these questions and I'll remember to give *The Complete Teething Guide* and Kathy the credit for my newfound expertise. I loved reading both the conventional discussions and the unusual theoretical parts of this book. I think you'll like it, too.

"It's just teething!"

Jay Gordon, MD, FAAP, IBCLC
Santa Monica, California

Introduction

Many people are unaware that our children's emotional and physical problems are often related to the teething process. Most equate "teething" with infancy, when it actually lasts through young adulthood. The teething process occurs in two phases. The first phase lasts from birth to 3 years – the period of time (weeks or months) preceding the eruption of a primary tooth, the process of it actually erupting and continues until the tooth finishes growing into position. This sequence of events repeats until all the primary teeth are in place. The second phase is from 5 years through adolescence – beginning with the movement of the unseen permanent teeth, continuing when a primary tooth becomes loose, losing the tooth, then cycling back to acquiring a whole new set of permanent teeth.

My main objective in writing this book was to help parents, doctors and school administrators have a better understanding of why our kids might be having trouble learning or concentrating (diagnosed as attention deficit hyperactivity disorder, ADHD or attention deficit disorder, ADD), are continuously sick, experience bouts of anxiety and depression, or are acting irrational and out of control.

Before my daughter was born I never imagined that teething would become part of my everyday vocabulary. Danielle was born in the winter of 1985, and from that moment on, we were caught in a teething frenzy, although we didn't know it at the time. Prior to that my only experience with children was babysitting as a teen and spending time with my two best friends' children. Their kids never seemed to have problems when they were teething.

My family was different: From the moment Danielle was born, her fist never left her mouth. When I look at pictures of our "mommy and me" group, there was never a photograph where Danielle didn't have her hand in her mouth. She was the wettest kid on the block, also known as the "drool queen." If she wasn't wearing a bib, her shirt was soaked from chin to waist. As a baby she would get blood blisters under the gum just before the eruption of a tooth, as well as most of the other symptoms described in this book.

As a first-time parent, I encountered many "firsts." With the arrival of Danielle's first tooth at 5 months came her first illness, which was addressed with antibiotic treatment. This was the beginning of what would become years of chronic health problems – croup, ear infections, enlarged tonsils, a suppressed immune system, nightmares, environmental stress, and food and chemical sensitivities, all compounded by repeated antibiotic use.

Danielle was also one of those statistics you are warned about when you vaccinate your child. She had a shock collapse syndrome at 18 months within three hours of being inoculated for diphtheria, pertussis (whooping cough), tetanus and polio, which is when I began to search for answers on how to rebuild her immune system. On my quest for better health, I was lead to information that was not readily available to the parenting mainstream. It quickly became evident to me that there were other families dealing with similar health problems, so in 1988, I started a newsletter, *Mother to Mother: Another View*, to help educate people about health and environmental issues and how they affect our children.

Over time, I began to recognize a synchronistic pattern to illness and behavior problems specific to certain age groups. I spent the next 15 years observing clients, friends and my daughter, researching the connection between teething, emotional behavior and physical symptoms.

Parents' personal experiences and stories continue to confirm my theories about the relationship between the teething process and a wide range of physical and emotional symptoms – fevers, drooling, headaches, diarrhea, vomiting, diaper rash, nightmares, sleeplessness, hyperactivity, trouble concentrating, teeth grinding, irrational, irritable or rhythmic behavior, fatigue, fears, anxiety, croup, depression, ear and/or throat problems, sinus congestion, a runny nose or even a cough. Clearly in the weeks, and sometimes months, preceding the eruption of a tooth, many infants and children experience a weakening of the immune system.

My observations suggest that seven out of 10 children come down with an illness or display suspicious emotional behavior prior to and during a tooth's eruption. My theory has raised many eyebrows and received quite a few chuckles. There is no scientific evidence to substantiate my findings, yet over the years, hundreds of parents have concurred with my conclusions.

Danielle is 18 years old now and still teething. She started getting her wisdom teeth when she was 15 1/2. So far, only two of them have partially broken through the gum. This three-year time span is testimony to the lengthiness of the teething process from start to finish. Her most recent symptoms include stomachaches, nausea, persistent cough, mood swings, irrational outbursts, irritability, croup, sinus congestion, and sleeplessness alternating with extreme fatigue. She also chews sugarless gum often because of a constant desire to chew on something. As you can see, teething is a long process and does continue through young adulthood.

Physical illness, especially in young children, is nothing to play with, or ignore and should be examined thoroughly, as well as treated responsibly. I have a great respect for the medical profession and the lifesaving miracles they can perform. But many parents are spending too much time at the doctor's office looking for a quick fix for the common cold, fever, flu, ear infections and more.

Twenty years ago, a parent was more apt to find answers to health-related questions through books written by respected pediatricians such as the late Benjamin Spock, M.D. Somehow the baby-boomer era brought with it much more dependent parents and frequent doctor visits. This increased need for pediatrician handholding has also encouraged the overuse of prescription drugs and created parents who have lost the ability to trust their instincts. The time has come to relearn this trust and combine it with old-fashioned common sense.

I am not a doctor or a dentist, but I am a mother who has spent the past 15 years researching all aspects of health, nutrition and teeth in relation to pregnancy, children, and adolescence. It is my honor to share this information with you through *The Complete Teething Guide: From Birth to*

Adolescence. I pray that this book will offer people new insights for better understanding a child's physical and emotional state. Please consider these ideas and observations as a different way of looking at things. The book is a compilation of the knowledge learned through personal experiences, observations, books, dentists, doctors and other health-care practitioners. I have tried to offer alternatives to traditional ways of thinking and, hopefully, open new doors in the field of dentistry. The information is not meant to take the place of or discourage parents from seeking professional medical advice or treatment when necessary. I hope it encourages you to speak up when something does not make sense, and teach you how to ask appropriate questions and get definitive answers from your doctor. It is empowering as parents when we realize that no one person has all the answers when it comes to the health and well-being of our children. Always contact your pediatrician or dentist with any questions, or in case of medical emergency, call 911.

Homeopathy

The homeopathic remedies referred to in this book are a therapeutic system of medicine developed by Samuel Hahnemann nearly 200 years ago in Germany. It is based upon the "law of similars" – "let likes be cured by likes". A homeopathic remedy is prepared by taking a minute dose of a substance – mineral, plant or animal, which if taken in large quantities would present a set of symptoms in the body. This substance is then diluted and made into a remedy that will stimulate and rebalance the immune system. An example is Ipecacuanha (Ipecac). The syrup of Ipecac is used to induce vomiting in case of accidental poisoning; when taken in homeopathic form of minute doses, it cures vomiting. The amount of times the substance is diluted determines the potency. For all reference in using homeopathic remedies in this book, the author suggests the 30X or 30C potency. If after three doses of a remedy the symptoms have not improved, consider changing the homeopathic medicine.

Flower Essences

The late Edward Bach, a scientist, bacteriologist and practicing physician, discovered flower essences in England back in the early 1930's. His research found that certain flower buds retain a vibration that can neutralize a negative emotion, returning the mental, physical and spiritual states back to balance. Bach originally formulated 38 different flower essences, but today there are thousands of other essences worldwide. The remedies are made from flowers' buds, clippings of wild bushes, plants and trees. Each essence is used to address a different emotion. An infusion is made in spring water and then usually preserved with alcohol. The remedy can be administered by adding a few drops of a stock bottle to another liquid beverage, placed directly onto the skin where it is absorbed into the body, or directly into the mouth. Since the flowers are absorbed through the skin, they can also be used in a humidifier, bath, soaking compress, etc. I generally avoid putting it directly into the mouth when working with newborns, infants or kids due to the alcohol content. Rescue Remedy or Five Flower essences are the most famous of the combination flower remedies. Both contain five different flower essence: Clematis – spacey or an unconscious state, Cherry Plum – feeling of being out of control (mind or body), Impatients – restoring patience, Rock Rose – panicky fear, Star of Bethlehem – loss, sorrow or grief. These two combination remedies are most commonly used in emergency or trauma situations.

Homeopathic and flower essence remedies are harmless and non-addictive; they have no side effects and will not interfere with other forms of alternative or traditional medicine. The remedies described in this book are considered safe and non-toxic for all ages. The four flower essence companies I refer to in the self-help sections throughout the book are: Bach/(B) • Botanical Alchemy/(BA) • Flower Essence Society/FES • Green Hope/(GH).

Even though the remedies are considered safe, the author and publisher disclaim all responsibility for any effects that may occur as a result of advice in context to this book. Always seek professional medical advise for any health or emergency related issues or call 911.

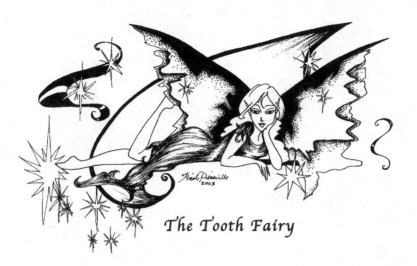

The Tooth Fairy

It is believed that the legend of the Tooth Fairy originated in either England or Ireland in the Middle Ages and was handed down over generations. As these myths evolved, they changed over the years and throughout the world. For instance, the Vikings had a "tooth fee," which was a form of reimbursement for using the child's teeth to make jewelry and was said to hold great powers and bestow good luck to the wearer. In some parts of Mexico, there is no tooth fairy at all, but a magic mouse that takes the tooth and leaves money. One American Indian tribe buries the tooth on the east side of a certain tree or bush, whereas another tribe may put it in a tree and then the family dances around it to insure the new tooth is strong and healthy. In other parts of the world, the child may throw the tooth on the roof, on the floor, over the bed, up to the sun, into the sea or bathtub, placed in a slipper, a box or even a glass of water, only to be retrieved by a mouse (for which there seems to be many different names), a different animal or a tooth fairy. Whatever the story, losing a tooth has a special meaning. And even if you don't believe in any of these legends, losing a tooth is still a milestone in a child's development, the transition from toddler to the next phase of childhood.

The tooth fairy lives in the land of your imagination. If you allow yourself to go to this magical place, you are afforded a special moment of sweet innocence. Many people don't believe in the tooth fairy, but for those who do believe, the preludes to each chapter are the creative efforts of some of my friends and have been contributed for your enjoyment. I would like to thank my young and not so young friends for sharing their beliefs and imaginations with us.

"*I believe the tooth fairy is the size of Tinker Bell, wears a long, flowing dress and has luminescent wings with sparkly dust on them that help her fly. She carries a small velvet bag filled with magic fairy dust, which when sprinkled over and around the children, offers pleasant dreams and special blessings. She also carries a magic wand. She can do almost anything with this wand, but most importantly it makes the exchange of tooth and gift without having to move the pillow. And just in case you were wondering what nationality this fairy is, well that too changes with a touch of the wand – she is multi-cultural. The wand also knows what the most appropriate gift should be for the child at hand, because each one is unique. The most common gift is money, but many children receive other treasures.*

I believe there is only one tooth fairy and that she lives in a tree castle in the forest where all her helpers, the other fairies and magical creatures live. Their surroundings are beautiful, with lots of brightly colored wild flowers, green lush vegetation and trees, deep, rich red soil and a slow moving-river cascading through the area. It is in this river where the teeth get their final cleaning. Once the dirt or plaque has been removed, the tooth is planted into the soil where the minerals are reabsorbed and used to feed and create new strong trees. Trees and teeth are similar in many ways. They start from tiny little buds or seeds and develop into layers or rings, known as "growth rings." These layers tell a story about their growth process. The layers of a tree can tell what kind of soil it was grown in or if it had a particularly hard winter. The layers of a tooth relay information such as what month a trauma, illness or nutritional deficiency may have occurred during the pregnancy. They both have roots that keep them firmly planted in their foundation – the soil or the gum tissue. It is amazing how much these two have in common."

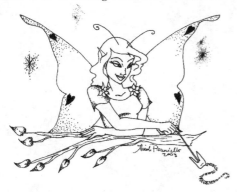

So, if your child has lost her first tooth today, whatever your beliefs are, be sure to honor the event and make it a special time.

Kathy
A mother's imagination

Chapter One

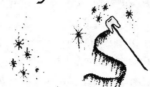

A Healthy Start: Building a Solid Foundation

Setting a solid foundation is essential for strong healthy teeth. When we begin to look at the delicate, intricate relationship between nutrition, illness, trauma and the development of teeth, it gives us a better understanding of the importance of these issues during pregnancy and the first years of life.

As a tree grows, it develops different layers called growth rings. These rings show a complete history of the tree itself – the type of soil it was grown in, its seasons, moisture quality and more. A tooth's developing process is similar to that of a tree's growth rings. During the fourth week of pregnancy, tiny cells are formed in the mouth of the fetus. These mature into different layers, better known as enamel and dentin, or "tooth rings." Enamel is the hard, white outer layer of the tooth and dentin is the softer layer under the enamel.

These tooth rings are a type of developmental map, which can be seen with the help of a microscope. The different layers reflect and record the development and history of a pregnant woman's health and nutrition, any trauma the unborn child may endure, as well as the health of a child in their early years. The rings are affected by factors such as a deficiency of certain nutrients, fevers, antibiotic use, too much fluoride, diseases, or even a difficult birth. Any of these incidences can influence the health, color and structure of a tooth.

Some conditions such as brain injuries can be traced back to an incident during a certain month of pregnancy by analyzing these tooth rings. The part of the tooth damaged or affected is dependent upon when the trauma occurred during its development. For instance, the brain of an infant with a type of childhood cerebral palsy (cerebral spastic infantile or Little's disease,) can be matched with specific tooth rings during the fifth month of pregnancy.[1] Teeth are imprinted with this knowledge for life.

◆ *Nutrition During Pregnancy* ◆

The time to start thinking about good nutrition and better health is long before you become pregnant. But, for many women today, pregnancy is the starting point to discover and learn about a healthier lifestyle.

I believe that nutrition in general is one of the most crucial aspects of one's physical and emotional health. However, this is a book on teeth and not specifically about nutrition, so I would like to encourage you to do further reading on nutrition for optimal health during pregnancy, breastfeeding, and for the newborn through adolescence. *(See recommended reading list.)*

According to the Food Science and Human Nutrition Department of Iowa State University, "Eating right, before and during pregnancy, can mean: fewer complications during pregnancy and delivery; less chance of birth defects; less chance of a premature baby; a stronger, healthier baby at birth; and a stronger you."[2]

From the moment of conception, your baby depends on the food you eat and the water you drink to supply energy, protein, vitamins, calcium, iron and other minerals and nutrients. Everything you do during pregnancy influences different aspects of your child's development and health. Your body has certain requirements to maintain good health, and once you become pregnant these needs increase. In addition to your own body's needs, you are now responsible for the nutritional needs of your developing baby.

• Tooth Development •

To give you a better understanding of the importance of good nutrition during pregnancy, let's take a closer look at the maturing process of a tooth. The course of a tooth's evolution actually takes place over years, starting in utero, continuing after birth, completing after eruption. In utero, growth of oral and facial structures occurs during the first four weeks of pregnancy. In the fifth week of an embryo's development, tooth formation begins with four buds on each side, top and bottom. Changes occur as each layer and part of the tooth is formed. As enamel cells grow and multiply, some of them become specialized creating the dentin and pulp. The enamel crowns of most of the baby teeth also start forming between the fourth and eighth week.[3]

The next phase of development is the calcifying, or hardening stage of the calcium salt in the teeth. In the ninth week, the enamel organ assumes the shape of a cap and by the fourteenth week, front teeth actually begin enamel development. This stage is completed between the first and second month after birth. Eruption of the primary teeth begins before the root is fully formed. The completed development takes place after the tooth's eruption.[4]

All the crowns of the baby teeth are formed after birth by the age of 12 to 15 months. The enamel doesn't start forming into the first permanent molars until shortly after birth. These molars begin erupting anytime between 4 1/2 and 7 years and are called, 6-year molars.[5] All 20 primary teeth, with the exception of the completed roots and mineralization process are formed in utero, which is why good nutrition during pregnancy is essential.

• Structure of the Teeth •

There are three main parts of a tooth – the *crown, neck and root*. What we see on top is the crown. The root is below the gum line and embedded in the bone. The point between the root and crown is the neck.

Enamel is the hardest substance in the body. It has been compared in strength and durability to the precious gem topaz.[6] Enamel by weight is composed of 96 percent inorganic minerals. The inorganic part is mainly calcium and phosphate. The remaining 4 percent consists of water and organic matter, mainly composed of a protein called keratin.[7] Enamel sits on the top of the tooth. It is not very thick, but still, it is the hardest of all tissues in the body. Enamel will wear with age from forceful biting or trauma.

Cementum is a bonelike substance that covers the roots of teeth. The fibrous tissues of the periodontal membrane are embedded in the cementum to allow the tooth to attach to the jaw. Cementum provides attachment for the fibers of the periodontal ligament, connecting the tooth securely to the alveolar bone of the tooth socket. When teeth are moved around with orthodontic devices, areas of cemental or root resorption can occur.

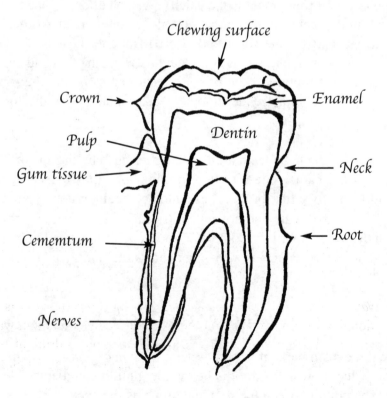

Tooth Structure

Dentin is tissue, which lies beneath the enamel and the cementum. It composes a greater bulk of the tooth. It is harder than cementum and softer than enamel. There are very fine nerve fibers in dentin, and it is a living tissue containing cells capable of repair. The hard tissue of both the crown and root contains 70 percent mineralized material and 30 percent organic portions and water. Dentin is softer and less resistant than enamel.

Pulp is the cavity that lies within the dentin. This cavity is filled with nerves, blood vessels and other soft tissue that attach in the jaw. This area reminds us that teeth are very much alive with nerves. It is divided into a canal and chamber. The small canal is in the center of the tooth, which has branches that go into the roots. This is the area that is involved in a root canal. The chamber is located in the center of the crown. Nerves in the pulp are responsible for the sensations we feel.[8]

Water, Complex Carbohydrates, Proteins & Fats

There are four basic nutritional components needed to maintain optimal health – water, complex carbohydrates, proteins and fats.[9]

◆ Water ◆

Water makes up approximately 70 percent of human body weight. It is responsible for the transportation of nutrients throughout the body, and plays a primary role in digestion, absorption, circulation and elimination. Thorough hydration is necessary for proper cell growth of the developing baby. According to F. Batmanghelidj, M.D., author of *Your Body's Many Cries for Water – You Are Not Sick, Just Thirsty*, morning sickness is the first indication that the embryo and mother are not receiving enough water during pregnancy. It is important for the average person to drink at least eight to 10 glasses of clean water a day, and during pregnancy, 10 glasses should be the minimum.

◆ *Carbohydrates* ◆

Starches are complex carbohydrates, and are found in whole grains, vegetables, legumes (dried beans, nuts, peas) and fruits; sugars are simple carbohydrates. The body gets energy from complex carbohydrates and needs them for digestion and the assimilation of food.

◆ *Protein* ◆

Proteins are composed of amino acids, which are the building blocks of human cells, and are essential for sustaining life. There are 22 primary amino acids, of which the human body can make only 14. The remaining eight (essential amino acids) need to be obtained through the diet. They are necessary for the production of hormones, antibodies, enzymes and the development of the nervous system.

All body tissue depends on sufficient amounts of protein. Protein provides a structural framework for the baby, including bones and teeth, the placenta, the production of breast milk, strengthening the uterus and healthy blood clotting.

There are two types of protein: complete and incomplete. Sources of complete proteins include milk, eggs, cheese, tofu or soybean products, fish, meat and poultry. Incomplete proteins are those missing certain amino acids and encompass whole grains, nuts, beans, peas and seeds. Incomplete proteins however, can be combined to achieve a complete protein status. For instance, beans or rice combined with nuts or seeds or simply the combination of beans and rice together all create a complete protein. *(See recommended reading list.)*

Low protein intake during pregnancy is associated with toxemia. Other symptoms associated with a protein deficiency include diarrhea, fatigue, vomiting and lack of appetite. Always consult a health care practitioner if any of these symptoms are present.

Opinions vary on how much protein is optimal during pregnancy. Some experts say 74 gm daily is sufficient, while others say a protein increase of

20 percent is what is needed. Lucy Moll, author of *The Vegetarian Child*, contends that getting enough protein is not an issue if a pregnant woman is eating enough calories from a variety of foods. In her book, Moll offers a simple formula for determining appropriate amounts of protein in general: Divide your weight in pounds by 2.2, which converts your weight into kilograms; then multiply that figure by 0.8. Based on this formula a 125-pound woman would require 46 gm of protein ($125 \div 2.2 = 57$ x $0.8 = 46$). According to the recommended daily allowance, a pregnant or nursing women would require an additional 10 to 15 gm of protein daily.[10] Another consideration to this equation is the individual's needs and ability to digest protein. Because of the broad scope of thought regarding protein intake during pregnancy, women should consult someone knowledgeable in this area, especially if you are a vegetarian.

Pregnant vegetarians should be eating at least five servings of fresh, organic vegetables and fruits a day. If a pregnant woman doesn't consume dairy products or eggs, she may substitute fortified products such as soymilk, cereals, etc., and take a B12 supplement, as this particular vitamin is found only in animal products.

◆ *Fats - Essential Fatty Acids (EFA)* ◆

For most, the word fat has negative connotations. The truth is there are "good" fats, or unsaturated fats, which are the polyunsaturated and monounsaturated fats (vegetable oils, cold-water fish, nuts and seeds), and "bad" fats, which are the saturated fats and trans-fatty acids or partially hydrogenated fats (margarine, chocolate, dairy, meat, processed foods). Good fats play an important role in the maintenance of good health.

Of the many known essential nutrients to the human diet, there are two essential fatty acids (EFAs) that are instrumental in producing omega-6 EFA, or arachidonic acid and omega-3 EFA or docosahexaenoic acid (DHA). These EFAs function as building blocks in membranes of every cell in the body. They produce prostaglandins, hormonelike substances necessary for energy production, fat metabolism, inflammatory response, blood pressure regulation, cardiovascular and immune function. DHA is also one of the most prevalent fats in the human brain and retina of the eye.[11]

Another area that DHA has proven to be of benefit is in regard to postpartum depression. During the last trimester of pregnancy the placenta depletes the mother's stores of DHA while passing them on to the fetus, as well as utilizing them in the production of breast milk. According to a National Institutes of Health study at Harvard University, there is a strong correlation between depression and lower levels of DHA.[12] With all of EFA's contribution, it is considered an important nutrient for a developing baby, a pregnant woman, and a breastfeeding infant's health.

We must get EFAs from our diet or supplementation because our bodies cannot make them. The World Health Organization suggests that EFAs make up 5 to 6 percent of a pregnant woman's daily caloric intake.[13] Typically, most people do not eat enough EFA-rich foods (certain nuts, seeds, oils and cold-water fish) to meet their daily requirements and supplementation is needed. Cold weather and winter months also increase the need for EFAs.

EFAs must be converted into other chemical forms. The body does this through a series of chemical reactions regulated by different enzymes. Enzymes depend on the presence of certain co-factor vitamins and minerals (i.e., B6, A, C, E, magnesium, zinc, copper and selenium) to help regulate proper EFA utilization. Sugar interferes with the process, which is another good reason to minimize your consumption of sugar during pregnancy. EFAs also reduce cholesterol and protect against heart disease.[14]

Water, complex carbohydrates, proteins and fats combined with other specific vitamins and minerals, are the foundation for proper growth and development, not only for the teeth but also for the overall health and well-being of the developing baby and pregnant woman.

During pregnancy, all nutrients are important, but special attention should be given to consuming foods rich in calcium, iron, zinc and folic acid. Ideally, we should be able to obtain proper nutrition by simply eating right, but today's typical American diet has more processed and contaminated foods than ever before. Processed foods contain preservatives, antibiotics, hormones, dyes, pesticides, artificial sweeteners, chemicals, stabilizers and some are even irradiated or genetically altered.

Unfortunately, all of these toxic foods have the potential to cause one or more of the following problems: cancer, neurotoxicity, birth defects, decreased immune function, food allergies and chemical reactions.[15] Purchase fresh organically grown fruits, vegetables, whole grains and legumes whenever possible. And for those who consume animal protein, free-range animal products raised without hormones, pesticides, antibiotics or chemicals will give you and your unborn baby the best advantage for optimal health and development.

◆ Vitamins & Minerals ◆

Vitamins and minerals are synergistic, which means there is a cooperative action between specific combinations. They act as catalysts, promoting the proper absorption and assimilation of each other. The vitamins and minerals listed work in unison to build stronger bones and teeth.

It is important to note that improper supplementation of certain nutrients during pregnancy can cause birth defects or stillbirths.[16] So, unless you are working with a trained professional, or are certain of what you are doing, beware of taking megadoses of vitamins individually, they can be risky.

Most obstetricians, midwifes and labor coaches suggest supplementing with a prenatal multivitamin-mineral to make sure all nutritional requirements are met. According to Arlene Eisenberg, Heidi Markoff and Sandee Hathaway, B.S.N., the authors of *What To Expect When You're Expecting*, "There are no standards set either by the FDA or by the American College of Obstetricians and Gynecologists specifying exactly what must be in a pill for it to be called a prenatal supplement."[17] Fortunately, most of the companies producing a more naturally based prenatal vitamin have done extensive research to provide a pregnant woman with an appropriate ratio of proper supplementation to be taken in conjunction with eating a healthful diet. But that does not mean a prenatal multivitamin-mineral will supply you with all the vitamins and minerals you will require on a daily basis. For instance, many women require more magnesium than is offered in most prenatal vitamins.

A good selection of prenatal vitamins can be found at your local natural foods market or holistic pharmacy. Look for one that contains no added binders, fillers, chemicals, dyes, sugar, corn, yeast or dairy. *(See resources in back of book.)*

◆ Minerals ◆

Calcium

Calcium is one of the most important minerals needed during pregnancy. It is found primarily in bones and teeth and considered to be one of the most plentiful minerals in the human body. Ninety-nine percent of calcium is found in bones and teeth with only 1 percent in the soft tissue.

Calcium is a mineral that continuously needs to be replaced and has a rhythm of movement. It is constantly being taken from the bones, moved out and used in other parts of the body, as well as being utilized by the unborn child. What is not being used is then excreted through the urine. If a mother's daily calcium intake is insufficient, her body will compensate by pulling calcium from her own bones and teeth to give it to the developing baby. This can put a woman at high risk for osteoporosis later in life.[18]

Phosphorus

Proper skeletal health however, requires more than just calcium. Phosphorus is another mineral, which is very instrumental in the teeth and bone equation. The delicate ratio between these two minerals is one of the main factors that determines the proper utilization of calcium in the body. The appropriate balance is believed to be 2:1 (calcium:phosphorus), the ratio found in breast milk.[19]

If there is too much calcium in the system it becomes non-functioning and will leave deposits or plaque on the teeth. If there is extra phosphorus, and the woman is not receiving enough calcium, it can present a negative calcium balance. If this happens, minerals are leached from the mother's bones, affecting both the teeth and bones of the woman and her developing baby.[20]

Unfortunately, with today's diet being what it is, the possibility of having too much phosphorus in the body is not uncommon. Foods that are high in phosphorus include many convenience foods, i.e., processed and snack foods, meats, cow's milk and carbonated beverages. Soft drinks or sodas are one of the biggest offenders of leaching minerals because they contain a substantial amount of phosphoric acid (phosphorus). If a pregnant woman drinks carbonated soda on a regular basis, she will most likely have too much phosphorus in her system, resulting in poor absorption of calcium, which can affect teeth and bone health. Foods that are high in calcium and low in phosphorus are vegetables, fruits and whole grains.[21]

Magnesium

The mineral magnesium is also important in at least a 2:1 (calcium:magnesium) ratio when taking a calcium supplement. Leo Galland, M.D., author of *Superimmunity for Kids*, suggests that some women may require twice as much magnesium or *equal* ratios to calcium, and in some cases more. Symptoms indicating a deficiency of magnesium include constipation, irritability, insomnia, headaches and premature uterine contractions. More severe consequences involve miscarriage, slow development and low birth weight of the infant.[22] A magnesium deficiency can also lead to the formation of kidney stones.

Magnesium is very important for the unborn baby. One West German study of 1,000 pregnant women found that those who supplemented with 400 mg of magnesium a day suffered less from toxemia, had fewer spontaneous abortions and delivered babies with higher birth weights and slightly higher Apgar scores.[23]

A woman should be receiving at least 450 mg of magnesium a day during pregnancy. The best supplemental forms are magnesium citrate or magnesium chloride. Naturally occurring magnesium can be found in nuts, legumes, whole grains, barley, dried fruits, honey and potatoes.

Besides a proper calcium, phosphorus and magnesium balance, additional factors that may inhibit the absorption and utilization of calcium include a deficiency of other minerals and vitamins, lack of sunlight exposure or vitamin D, hormones and consuming excess amounts of protein, sugar, caffeine or high-sodium foods. Too much protein in the diet will cause a loss of calcium because the body does not store the excess, but excretes it through the urine, taking with it important minerals.

Many pregnant women do not realize how important calcium intake is for their developing baby, and assume their prenatal multivitamin and mineral will give them all they need. Unfortunately, that is not the case. The National Institutes of Health recommends that pregnant women get 1,500 mg of calcium a day, but many prenatal vitamins only have 250 mg.

Some studies show that it isn't necessarily how much calcium you are consuming, but rather, how much is actually being absorbed that is important. One study in rural China found that the Chinese, who consume far less calcium than Americans, seemed to have less osteoporosis. A key factor in this finding is that the Chinese consume far less protein than most Americans.[24]

Health researcher and writer Mark Lovendale notes the results of another study funded by the dairy industry in 1985, in which three different groups of young women were followed. Women in Group I drank three additional glasses of milk a day and lost twice as much calcium from their bones. Those in Group II consumed an average amount of dairy products and still lost bone calcium. Yet the women in Group III who were on a low-protein, diary-free diet, experienced no calcium loss at all.[25]

Another advantage of having adequate amounts of calcium in the body is that it protects the body by inhibiting its absorption of lead. Over the years, lead is stored in the body as a result of different exposures such as lead pipes, water, paint, etc. If the mother-to-be is not receiving enough calcium in her diet, it can cause this stored lead to be dispersed into the bloodstream and affect both the mother and her unborn baby.[26] Ninety percent of the lead stored in the mother's body is free to cross the placenta, which then becomes available for deposit in the bones and teeth of the developing baby. This release of lead also puts the pregnant woman at risk by causing an increased rate of miscarriages and stillbirths.

Different symptoms that may indicate a woman is suffering from a calcium deficiency during pregnancy are muscle cramps, backache, intense labor and afterbirth pains, teeth problems, high blood pressure and preeclampsia, a condition portrayed by acute high blood pressure, edema and excessive protein loss in the urine.

According to a study conducted by the World Health Organization (*British Medical Journal*, August 1997), research suggests, it may even be possible to actually program a child's blood pressure for life by supplementing extra calcium during pregnancy. The authors of current studies suspect that the extra calcium either directly affects the mechanisms regulating blood pressure or influences the way the child's cardiovascular system develops. Still more studies are needed to confirm these conclusions.[27]

There are many good sources of calcium available from the foods we eat, least of which are dairy products. Years ago, a major advertising campaign was conducted by milk producers with the slogan, "Everybody needs milk." This strong media influence was instrumental in convincing the American public that dairy products are responsible for providing us with a majority of our calcium requirements, even though the industry never actually came out and said that.[28]

In 1974, the Federal Trade Commission issued a 'proposed complaint' citing the slogan as misleading. But, by this time, people were already convinced that if they were not consuming milk or cheese products, their bones would be doomed.[29]

According to Frank Oski, M.D., author of *Don't Drink Your Milk*, one quart of cow's milk contains 1,200 mg of calcium, as compared to human milk, which only has 300 mg per quart. Interestingly enough, he states, "The infant receiving the human milk actually absorbs more calcium into his body."[30]

Mark Lovendale also states, "The high phosphorus level in dairy products causes dairy calcium to be poorly assimilated as compared to the calcium from vegetables. People who are free of dairy products and other allergy causing foods, while avoiding a high protein diet, have strong bones and receive all the calcium they need from a full range of vegetables."[31]

Calcium-Rich Foods

Corn bread - 1 two-ounce piece = 133 ml
Dried figs (10) = 269 ml.
Nuts, almonds and hazelnuts 1/4 cup = 100-200 ml
Sesame seeds, 1 tablespoon = 125 ml
Raw firm tofu, 1/2 cup = 258 ml

Boiled vegetables - 1 cup each:
Broccoli – 178 ml, kale = 94 ml
Butternut squash = 84 ml
Sweet potato = 70 ml

Boiled beans - 1 cup each:
Great Northern = 121 ml
Navy = 128 ml
white = 161ml
Pinto = 82 ml
Vegetarian baked = 128 ml
Chickpeas, canned = 78 ml

Sea vegetables:
Kombu, nori and wakame, 1 tablespoon = 100-200 ml

Fish, such as salmon and sardines, are also good sources. These are just some of the many foods that contain calcium.[32, 33]

Herbal sources of calcium include alfalfa, red clover, red raspberry leaves, nettle, chamomile, dandelion, kelp and dulse.[34] Tori Hudson N.D., author of *Woman's Encyclopedia of Natural Medicine*, suggests raspberry leaf tea, nettle tea, fresh parsley and watercress as the most absorbable forms of calcium.[35]

In terms of a calcium supplement, the most easily absorbed forms are calcium citrate or citrate/malate. These have been found to be most effective when taken in small doses of 500-600 mg over the course of a day, rather than in a megadose all at once.[36] Be sure to drink a lot of water. Calcium supplements to avoid during pregnancy include dolomite, bone meal and oyster shell because of the high lead content as well as other toxic metals.[37]

Zinc

Zinc is another important mineral for the development of an unborn child. The requirements will increase during pregnancy, as the placenta is the richest source of zinc there is. Depending on its size, the placenta will contain between 300-600 mg of zinc.[38]

Zinc is essential in the development of skeletal muscle and bones, before and after birth; for brain formation and functioning; and is instrumental in giving connective tissue elasticity. Even though there are no statistics, it has been said that this mineral can help prevent stretch marks, tearing of the perineum and cracks in the breast tissue during nursing. A woman who is lacking zinc in her diet may have white spots on the fingernails, a prolonged labor and compromised uterine membrane contractions. Zinc deficiencies have also been linked to fetal growth retardation, congenital defects, undescended testes, excessive crying and inconsolable, jittery infants.[39]

Inorganic iron and calcium interfere with the absorption of zinc, so it is best to take the mineral on an empty stomach. The recommended dosage of zinc during pregnancy is 20 mg. This figure will increase again during breastfeeding.[40]

There is a zinc taste test to help determine appropriate zinc levels. Most natural food stores carry a solution called zinc sulphate. To test your zinc levels, simply swish one teaspoon in your mouth. Different taste responses will give you a good indication as to where your zinc levels stand. If the taste is extremely unpleasant, your levels are fine. Be prepared to spit out the solution quickly if necessary.

Some foods that contain plentiful amounts of zinc include egg yolks, brewer's yeast, lima beans, liver, pecans, pumpkin seeds, sardines, soybeans, sunflower seeds, lamb chops, meat, pecans, walnuts and rye.

◆ *Vitamins* ◆

Vitamin A

Vitamin A is a fat-soluble vitamin that acts as a strong antioxidant for the immune system. Despite its benefits, it can also be dangerous and toxic when taken in large quantities. Excessive supplementation during pregnancy can cause permanent fetal malformation or birth defects.[41] On the other hand, a deficiency of this vitamin has been linked to premature birth, miscarriage and lung problems, as well as abnormalities in the newborn, such as cleft palate and no eyes.[42]

Most experts agree that when taken in supplemental form, vitamin A intake should not exceed 6,000IU per day while pregnant. If you are taking a prenatal vitamin you are most likely already meeting this limit.

Some prenatal vitamin manufacturers now use a non-toxic beta-carotene, which is a precursor to the fat-soluble vitamin A. This form of A is derived from plant sources like yellow and orange fruits and vegetables. For example, carrot juice and sweet potatoes are high in beta-carotene. Carotenoids are most effective when they are mixed, but should not exceed dosages higher than 10,000IU a day during pregnancy. Herbal sources include alfalfa, dandelion, elderberries and seaweed.[43]

Vitamin C (Ascorbic Acid) with bioflavonoids

Vitamin C is a strong antioxidant that protects the body from invading viruses, bacteria and environmental pollutants, it is needed for the production of collagen, a protein needed for forming connective tissue in skin, ligaments and bones of the developing baby, as well as the expanding mother-to-be.

Vitamin C also aids in the proper assimilation and utilization of other minerals and vitamins important for growing bones and teeth, such as calcium, magnesium, iron, folic acid and vitamins A and D. I prefer the Ester-C mineral ascorbate with bioflavonoids. Studies have shown that this unique form of vitamin C is transported into the bloodstream faster, in larger amounts, is held there longer, and penetrates white blood cells more efficiently, making it the most bioavailable form developed.[44] It is also ph neutral, which makes it easier on the stomach.

According to Jill Romm, author of *The Natural Pregnancy Book,* the dosage of vitamin C should not exceed 2,000 mg a day during pregnancy. She cautions, "It can lead to miscarriage in early pregnancy and can cause a vitamin C dependency in the baby which can lead to scurvy in a newborn."[45]

Vitamin D

Vitamin D is another vitamin that helps metabolize calcium. The best natural source of vitamin D is sunlight. Other sources are fish oil and the herbs alfalfa and nettles. Further supplementation of vitamin D should only be done under the advice of a professional because excessive amounts of the vitamin can be toxic and cause the same symptoms as excessive sun exposure – nausea and dizziness.

The key to good nutrition during pregnancy is learning to eat right so that you will receive the most benefits out of what you are putting into your body.

✦ Nutrition for Children ✦

Getting children to eat healthily is a real challenge today, with every other commercial on television promoting fast food or junk food. Most advertised foods are laced with sugar, chemicals, preservatives and dyes, and have been irradiated, genetically modified or contain growth hormones.

Just as a pregnant woman's nutritional habits will affect her unborn child's developing teeth, the general eating habits of an infant, young child and adolescent will affect their teeth. Introducing foods that support a balanced diet as early as possible helps build strong, healthy bones and teeth.

◆ Newborn - 6 months ◆

The optimal form of proper nutrition for a newborn to the age of 6 months is supplied through breast milk. Even the American Academy of Pediatrics recommends that breast milk be an infant's main source of nutrition for the first year. Solids should not be introduced until after six months because until then babies lack certain enzymes responsible for proper digestion.

Mother's milk is nature's perfect formula. It supplies appropriate ratios of vitamins, minerals, amino acids, good bacteria, immunoglobins and interferon, all of which contribute to protecting an infant against a wide range of infections and viruses. Breast milk also contains enzymes that break down fat in milk to form individual free fatty acids, which inhibit the growth of parasites in the intestines that can cause diarrhea. There are at least 10 hormones in breast milk that help regulate growth, metabolism and maturation of the intestine and other body tissues. Another important contribution is lactoferron, a protein that combines with iron and makes it easier to absorb, again inhibiting the growth of bacteria.

Not all women are able to breastfeed their newborns. Some women simply aren't interested, whereas others may have physical limitations, need to return to work, or have adopted the baby. Whatever the reason for not breastfeeding, the next best choice is supplementing with a naturally based infant formula. To date, I know of only one company that offers an organic formula, Nature's One. Their Baby's Only Organic pediatric formula is made with either a dairy or soy base. Both formulas can be used as an infant formula under the guidance of a health-care professional that best understands the baby's specific needs.

During the first few months, an infant's body goes through a transition of integrating its new method of consuming nutrition orally and the elimination process. This is a time of learning for both baby and parent. A newborn's immature digestive system will respond in different ways through this adjustment period. The most common problematic symptoms a baby may experience during this stage are constipation, gas, cramping, fussiness, spitting up and, in some cases, vomiting.

If any of these symptoms do arise, generally speaking, the process of figuring out what works best for you and your baby will be an experiment. If you are breastfeeding, you might need to eliminate certain foods from your diet to remedy the situation. If you are using infant formula, you may have to try a few different brands before you find the one your baby will tolerate best.

If a baby becomes fussy during the night, many parents assume that the infant is hungry and worry that breast milk or formula is not enough nourishment to sustain them. This idea offers a temptation to start solid food earlier with the hope of remedying sleepless nights. One study between two separate groups of 6-week-old infants, showed no change in sleep habits when they were supplemented with infant cereal. One group was fed rice cereal before bed and the other group was not given anything. The results from this study help put to rest the theory that solid food helps an infant sleep through the night.[46] *(See chapter on "Breastfeeding and Bottle-Feeding.")*

◆ 6 - 12 months ◆

The first solid food usually offered to an infant is iron-fortified cereal – rice, oat or barley. During the first 6 months, an infant will receive all the iron they need from breast milk or formula in a form that is easy to absorb. But as you introduce solid food, this form of iron becomes harder to assimilate and supplementation will be needed. Iron helps support proper brain development and the production of white blood cells for a healthy immune system. A deficiency of iron can cause anemia and increase a child's absorption of lead from food, which can adversely affect their intellectual function.[47]

Ways to supplement iron once foods are introduced include iron-fortified foods; preparing foods in cast-iron pans; a liquid infant multivitamin; and foods such as apricots, peaches, pears, avocados, peas, pumpkin, dates, whole grains, tofu and dulse, a sea vegetable. Dairy products inhibit the absorption of iron and vitamin C-rich foods enhance it.

If the child is diagnosed with anemia, ferrous sulfate or an herbal iron can be supplemented, but only under the guidance of a health-care practitioner. The reason it is important to work with a doctor is that an excess of supplemental iron can be dangerous and toxic if not administered properly, especially for an infant.

If you are breastfeeding, it is important to remember not to let solid food come first, always offer the breast before a meal. This practice will ensure a continued proper caloric intake as well as an adequate nutrient balance.

The longer you wait to introduce food, the less chance there will be of a child developing an allergy. When a child starts eating solid food, the protective *Lactobacillus bifidus* in his intestines will start to disappear, so the later you start solids the stronger the immune system will be. There are many foods that can stimulate an allergic reaction and should be avoided during the first year. These foods are corn, tomato, egg, honey, wheat, citrus fruit, milk, chocolate, fish, strawberries and nuts. Peanuts, although called a nut, are actually the pod of a plant of the legume family. They are another highly allergenic food that really shouldn't be given to children under the age of two or even three years.[48] Honey can cause botulism in infants because they do not have the enzymes adults have to break it down. Also, a low-protein diet is best for the first year, as a young digestive system can have trouble assimilating it.

According to Peggy O'Mara, author of *Natural Family Living – The Mothering Magazine Guide to Parenting*, signs of physical readiness for the introduction of solid foods include: being able to sit up, the infant losing his tongue-thrusting reflex (which pushes the food back out, rather than allowing it to be swallowed), and manual dexterity to pick up food and bring it to the mouth.

Introduce one food at a time to help detect food allergies or sensitivities. Start with a spoonful and remember less is better in the beginning. Give the same food for at least three days and watch for signs of an allergy. Any of the following symptoms fall into this category – rash, hives, breathing problems, congestion, constipation, gas/abdominal cramps, diarrhea and fussiness.

If you do encounter a problem, eliminate the food. If it is a mild reaction, try reintroducing the food in a month or two. If there is a strong reaction, be sure to notify your child's doctor as well as any caregivers. That way, everyone responsible for the infant/child's safety will be well informed. For severe reactions, such as anaphylactic shock (a swelling in the throat and/or a restriction of the airways), call 911 immediately.

There are different thoughts on which food should be introduced next, fruits or vegetables. Leo Galland, M.D., encourages pureed, cooked vegetables as the succeeding food. He suggests peas, green beans, sweet or white potato, squash or pumpkin, rotating one new food every three or four days. Susan Roberts, Ph.D., Melvin Heyman, M.D. and Lisa Tracy, authors of *Feeding Your Child for Lifelong Health*, suggest a more traditional start with pureed cooked apple, pear, peach, prune or raw ripe mashed banana as the next palate pleaser. After 8 or 9 months the baby will enjoy other fruits and vegetables such as avocado, papaya, zucchini, etc.

One thing these authors agree on is if you are preparing your infant's vegetables from scratch, stay away from vegetables that are rich in natural nitrates such as spinach, beets, turnips, carrots, string beans and collard greens, until after the age of 9 months. Galland states, "Nitrates can change red blood cells so that they are less able to carry oxygen."[49] Nitrates are converted to nitrites in an immature digestive system and can cause a life-threatening form of anemia called methemoglobinemia.[50] Baby food companies buy their produce from areas where nitrate levels are low, and have a screening process to monitor the levels in their commercially made baby food to make sure the vegetables are safe for infants. If you are using store-bought baby food be sure to look for organic, non-irradiated brands with no added sugar or salt. This will give your baby the best possible start.

Once the baby is 10 months old, their digestive tracts and kidneys are ready to handle some protein. You can start with small portions of pureed cooked lean beef or poultry, tofu, soy products, beans, etc. Remember to keep the rotation schedule of one new food every three or four days, and continue the observation process for food sensitivities and/or allergies.

◆ 12 months - Early Childhood ◆

After 12 months, as the diet becomes more diverse, there are special considerations pertinent to the proper assimilation of a child's nutrients in the development of strong bones and teeth. In today's society, most children are malnourished, not obviously by sight, but recognized through hair, skin, teeth, behavior, illness, learning ability and more. Our job is to teach our kids to enjoy foods that will promote healthy, long-term development.

In *Feeding Your Child for Lifelong Health*, the authors describe the new science of "Metabolic Programming" or MP. MP is a new term, which describes how foods eaten in early childhood can have lasting effects on the way a child's body grows and functions. The authors state, "Scientists believe that MP happens in part because growth and cell division in many parts of the body occur only in childhood. During this time, individual cells are sensitive to the availability of nutrients."

It appears that early childhood offers this special window of opportunity for building a solid foundation for long-term permanent effects on intelligence, weight balance, growth, strength (including bones and teeth), blood pressure and overall immune system function.

Children have different nutritional needs than adults. They need more fat and less fiber. Many parents are unaware of these differences and become consumed with their own diets of low-fat or no-fat in order to stay trim, never realizing this diet can be harmful for their infant or young child. A newborn requires 50 percent of his calories from dietary fat to support proper growth and development. This percentage decreases over time to about 30 percent by the age of 3 years.

More on Fats - Essential Fatty Acids (EFAs)

The reason fats are so important in the first few years, is because most brain tissue is formed after birth. The brain is 60 percent fat by weight. An infant has 30 percent the number of brain cells as an adult. The growth process is so fast in these first few years that by 12 months, brain development will reach 90 percent and by 18 months, 95 percent of its full potential.

In order to support your infant's body nutritionally during this period of brain growth, it is important to supplement the diet with essential fatty acids. The two most valuable essential fatty acids are docosahexaenoic acid (DHA) or omega-3 and arachidonic acid or omega-6 oils. These are the good fats that the body needs to develop optimally. The body will require an additional source of EFAs because it cannot make its own, nor can it get enough from the foods we eat.

These good fats are unsaturated fats, obtained from vegetable oils, cold-water fish, nuts and seeds. These unsaturated fats contribute to proper brain and eye development, hormone regulation, cardiovascular function, fat metabolism, and inflammatory response, immune and nervous system function.

If you are nursing, the infant will receive all the EFAs needed through nature's perfect source. However, mom should be supplementing her diet with additional amounts of EFAs to keep up with both of their requirements.

If the infant is drinking formula, you can easily include a plant-based supplement such as flaxseed oil or perilla oil into the bottle. If for some reason your baby doesn't like the taste of the oil in the formula, it can actually be massaged directly into her skin. Both ways are effective in supplying the extra EFA an infant will need. (Hemophiliacs should use caution in the use of EFA in general, due to its blood thinning properties.)

As you introduce solids, the flaxseed oil or powder, or perilla oil can be added to an infant's food. In order to maintain the stability of the oil, do not microwave formula or foods containing flaxseed or perilla oil. Never use the oil for frying or sautéing as the combination of high heat and oxygen destroys its EFAs. It should be stored in the refrigerator to preserve its freshness. Both of these oils and the flax powder have a fairly pleasant taste. If it has a rancid taste or smell, throw it away. A child may show signs of an EFA deficiency by being thirsty all the time, lacking hair luster, dry brittle nails or a skin rash on various parts of the body. Always consult a qualified source to help determine appropriate amounts for your baby's individual needs.

Children will require much less fiber than an adult. There are literally no fiber recommendations for children under the age of one year. The digestive system is immature and still does not have the ability to fully process fiber. An old standard set by the American Academy of Pediatrics Committee on Nutrition suggests that an appropriate fiber recommendation can be determined by calculating the age plus 5g. So, between the ages of 1 and 3 years, the suggested fiber range is 6-8g and between 4 and 6 years 9-11g. Teens between the ages of 13 and 15 years need 18-20g and 16 to 19-year-olds need 21-24g. The recommendation for an adult is from 25-30g. As you can see there is quite a difference in the diet structures of an infant, child, adolescent and adult.

Appropriate calorie intake is another area of interest when it comes to children. Calories are a measure of energy found in all foods, particularly those with high amounts of carbohydrates or fat. Everyone needs a certain amount of calories per day to sustain energy and grow properly. I frequently receive calls from distressed parents concerned about their child's lack of interest in food. When a child is teething, different symptoms may arise, one of them being a loss of appetite. (Be sure to always investigate other possibilities for this absence of hunger.) The good news is authors Roberts, Heyman and Tracy suggest that current research supports a 15 percent decline in the amount of calories necessary to maintain proper nutritional balance. So rest assured, children can actually survive on fewer calories, providing they are productive calories and not empty ones full of sugar. For a 3-month-old, the average calorie intake is approximately 550 calories; 1 year – 850; 2 years – 1,050; 3 years – 1,250 and for a 6-year-old – 1,550. These averages will also depend on the child's size, weight, activity level and overall constitution.[51]

When we examine the diet of young children, we are faced with the reality of many adversities and myths. Most children watch television and are greatly influenced (as are their parents) by the advertisements for cereal, dairy, meats, processed foods, etc. and the restaurants serving them. These foods are high in saturated fats (which are bad fats), filled with sugar and full of chemicals, pesticides, preservatives and colored dyes. They are also high in sodium and include foods made with genetically engineered or irradiated ingredients.

♦ Minerals For Children & Adolescents ♦

I feel the mineral component is essential to all phases of development and would like to reaffirm the information presented in the earlier section for pregnancy with regard to growth requirements for young children and adolescents. The principal minerals for building strong teeth and bones are calcium, phosphorus, magnesium, zinc and iron. Mineral absorption and utilization is the key to achieving this strong foundation.

There are several contributing factors that run interference in the mineral assimilation process – diets which are high in sodium, phosphorus, saturated fats, protein, sugar, and caffeine.

The ratio and balance of these minerals together are what determines whether or not, they are used properly by the body. For instance, calcium needs a 2:1 ratio with phosphorus. This is probably the hardest mineral ratio to balance with today's diet structure. Food sources that are high in phosphorus include dairy, carbonated beverages (sodas), meats, and processed convenient snack foods. When there is not enough calcium, and the phosphorus levels are too high, the missing minerals will be leached directly from a child's bones. The consequences of this mineral depletion are usually undetectable until later in life with osteoporosis or tooth loss. However, one of my daughter's girlfriends was addicted to carbonated soda, which is high in phosphorus. She was drinking one to three cans of soda a day, with the rest of her diet consisting of a fair share of diary products, also high in phosphorus. Between the age of 12 and 15 years, this young lady suffered repeated breaks to her bones in different areas of her body.

The metabolic signals for calcium absorption begin at birth and will continue through adolescence. This is a crucial period of time when essential calcium is deposited in the bones and teeth and will establish strength and health for life.

The dairy industry and media have been very influential in convincing the American public that by consuming milk and cheese, appropriate calcium requirements will be achieved. Unfortunately, dairy is an over publicized food source with the potential for a list of nutritional imbalances. Diary products are a major source of saturated fat and produce high cholesterol levels. One report in the *New England Journal of Medicine* in 1992 by Dr. Han-Michael Dosch, showed support for the theory that cow's milk proteins stimulate the production of the antibodies which in turn, destroy the insulin-producing pancreatic cells. Evidence suggests that the combination of a genetic predisposition and the exposure to cow's milk is the major cause of childhood diabetes. Unfortunately, there is no way of determining which children are genetically predisposed to this condition. Antibodies form in response to even small quantities of milk products, including infant formulas. Charles Attwood, M.D., author of *Dr. Attwood's Low-Fat Prescription for Kids* states, "Other scientists have also noted and reported since 1990, that more diabetes is found in countries where people consume the most milk."[52]

In many cases, iron deficiency anemia is also produced by an allergy to the protein in cow's milk. Fifteen to 20 percent of the children in the U.S. suffer from iron deficiency anemia. Some infants' sensitivities to cow's milk result in a slow and steady bleeding which is lost through the stool and undetectable to the naked eye. According to Frank Oski, M.D., author of *Don't Drink Your Milk!*, it is estimated that half the cases of this form of anemia among infants in the United States are the result of gastrointestinal bleeding prompted by cow's milk. Symptoms to watch for include irritability, apathy, fatigue, and inattentiveness.[53]

Zinc deficiencies are also likely to occur in kids who eat a lot of cheese and drink milk. Galland suggests that young children who receive most of their nutrition from milk and cheese are prone to a deficiency of zinc. Zinc is essential because it controls processes that only take place during childhood, such as cell division, growth, and protein synthesis. A deficiency may express itself through a weakened immune system, irritability, stunted growth, or jittery nerves.

Saturated fats (hydrogenated or partially hydrogenated oils) are found in margarine, chocolate, dairy, meat, and processed foods. These fats are responsible for fatty deposits in the coronary arteries of children as young as 3-years-old. Attwood also suggests that by the age of 12 years, nearly 70 percent of the children are affected by these early stages of heart disease, and states, "More advanced deposits rapidly appear throughout the teens."

If a child is eating the wrong types of fats (saturated) and not getting enough of certain essential vitamins and minerals, the body cannot make proper use of the EFAs, which are responsible for regulating hormone levels. Butter vs. margarine – according to the technical support team at Omega Nutrition, moderate consumption of (unsalted) butter in conjunction with unrefined vegetable oils is an excellent source of food energy. Butter can be directly utilized by the body and requires no liver conversion whereas margarine is a hydrogenated, high-temperature refined vegetable oil, which produces a poisonous molecular change in trans-fatty acids and is difficult for the body to process.

Weston Price, D.D.S., author of *Nutrition and Physical Degeneration*, established that butter concentrate increased mineral absorption to support healthier bones and teeth. He credits an unknown fat substance in butter to be responsible for stimulating bone growth. A colleague of Prices, Hal Huggins, D.D.S., found that he could tell if a child was raised on butter or margarine by their facial form and tooth's position.[54]

Another concern with regard to having enough calcium in the body is that it inhibits the absorption of lead. If a child is deficient in calcium, lead that is stored accumulatively in the body over years is then released into the bloodstream. Once this lead is disbursed, it is absorbed by the body and deposited in the teeth and bones. This could account for higher levels of lead in children who are more prone to cavities. In January of 1990, The *New England Journal of Medicine* cited a study which suggests, "Low levels of lead in children may lead to lifelong problems such as severe reading problems, poor eye-hand coordination, slower reflexes, and hyper-activity."[55]

The magnesium ratio to calcium is also very important for young children. Pediatrician Paul Fleiss, M.D., feels magnesium is an abundant mineral, yet the most neglected nutrient in this category. Many nutritional formulas only have a 2:1 calcium:magnesium ratio, but now pediatricians are suggesting that more is needed. Equal ratios of calcium and magnesium are much more adequate for the stresses of our children today, not in terms of proper assimilation of calcium, but rather in regard to bodily functions. A child who is deficient in magnesium may be constipated, irritable, or have trouble sleeping and suffer from chronic headaches.

Conclusion

If your children eat a variety of fresh fruits and vegetables, eggs, fortified foods, fish, meat, poultry, soy protein and whole grains, and take a natural multivitamin-mineral supplement, they will be receiving plenty of these vital nutrients. The only additional requirements they may need are the mineral magnesium and essential fatty acids or EFAs. Keep in mind that if the child is eating a diet low in saturated fats, sodium, phosphorous, protein and sugar, they will absorb their nutrients more efficiently.

Vitamins that are key elements in the teeth and bone equation are vitamins A, B, C and D (sunlight).

Vitamin A
- An important vitamin in the formation of bones and teeth.
- A deficiency produces poor enamel quality that is rough and decays easily.
- A deficiency can produce an irregular band on the tooth. This is true for both vitamin A and D.
- A deficiency can be associated with abnormal tooth and bone formation.
- A deficiency will cause infections to heal slowly.
- Teens whose diets consist of meat, potatoes and fast foods, are usually lacking in vitamin A. (Vitamin A can be toxic if taken in large doses over a period of time).

B vitamins

- A deficiency produces an increased susceptibility to decay.
- A deficiency increases the severity of gingivitis (inflammation of the gums).
- Sores at angles of the mouth with chapped, cracked lips can signify a deficiency.
- Red, painful tongue, and small ulcers on gums can be from a deficiency.
- A deficiency can lead to trench mouth (an acute ulcerating infection of the gums and throat).

Vitamin C

- An antioxidant which aids in calcium absorption.
- A deficiency can cause gums to swell and bleed (in some cases profusely) during tooth eruption.
- A deficiency accelerates destructive effects of inflammation on bone.
- A deficiency can cause severe gingivitis (inflammation of the gums) in teens.
- An increased susceptibility to infection and slower healing, are also signs of a deficiency.

Vitamin D

- Helps build strong jawbones and teeth.
- A deficiency creates problems in the enamel and eventual deterioration of the bone structures in the jaw.
- A severe vitamin D deficiency is called Rickets.
- Sunlight exposure is the best source of this nutrient.

"My tooth fairy looks cute and she is tall. She feels real soft and she acts like an angel to everyone. She is a girl and her name is Candy. Her hair is black and a bit of brown. Oh yeah, there is one more thing, she could fly high and do magic. She flies by using magical powers because the master gave her the powers. When she got her powers was June 1, 2002 and she got them in the courtroom. She needs lots of power for her wand to change the tooth into a half dollar. She got her wings when she passed her test and she got her wand when she was ready. Now you know all about her."

Ana - 8 years old

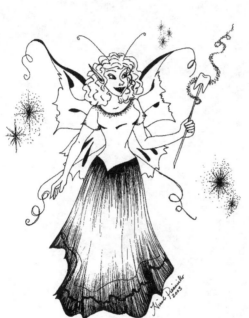

"I lost only one tooth so far. It was really wiggly and I was at a pool party and it fell out and got lost. I had to write the tooth fairy a note and tell her what happened. It must have been okay because she gave me some money. But I didn't see her because she is invisible. She walks right through the window to get into my house when I am sleeping. She takes the tooth and adds it to her house where she makes them into necklaces and money. She lives in a castle in the sky with all the other fairies. There are girl fairies – they bring the things for the girls and there are boy fairies – they bring the money to the boys."

Rachel - 6 years old

Chapter Two

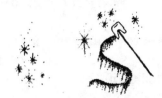

A Teething Timeline

• Natal & Neonatal Teeth •

Sometimes a baby is born with a visible tooth or teeth – this is very rare, but it does happen. These teeth are called natal teeth. It is not uncommon for a natal tooth to have an underdeveloped root causing the tooth to be loose. When this happens, a dentist may recommend the tooth be extracted because of the risk of choking. However, I would always suggest getting a second or third opinion before allowing a dentist to pull a natal tooth. Keep in mind a natal tooth is also a primary tooth and helps guide a secondary tooth to its proper position. Discuss all the risks and options with your dentist or doctor.[1]

Self-help:
There are two good homeopathic remedies that can be used to try and stabilize a weak root system of a natal tooth: *Calcarea fluorica* – when a tooth is loose in the socket; and *Calcarea Phosphorica* – can help restore tone to weakened tissue and is an essential constituent in the formation of teeth. These two remedies can be used together in a 6x potency.[2] The best way to administer a homeopathic remedy to a newborn is by using the soft tablets and putting 1-2 drops of water on them. They will dissolve instantly and you can scoop up the paste on your finger and put it directly in the infant's mouth. (Always consult an educated practitioner with your specific questions.)

A neonatal tooth is a tooth that erupts after birth. It is usually much stronger than a natal tooth, even if it erupts in the first month, right after birth.[3]

◆ *Deciduous & Succedaneous Teeth* ◆

The first set of teeth has several different names – baby teeth, milk teeth, primary teeth or deciduous teeth. Deciduous comes from the Latin word *decidere*, which means "to fall off" or shed. The word "primary" represents first in order, or in this case, a first set of teeth.

Most children have 20 primary teeth – 10 upper (maxillary) and 10 lower (mandibular) showing by the age of 3. The primary teeth are important for learning how to talk, helping the jaw grow to its proper shape and size, and guiding the permanent teeth to their proper position.

The transition of shedding the primary teeth begins sometime between the ages of 5 and 7 years, and continues through the ages of 12 to 14 years. The first tooth to fall out is most often a central incisor, as the adult tooth pushes upward. This process is usually concurrent with the eruption of the first permanent molar (6 year molar) on the same side and location (upper or lower, left or right), but again, this is not always the case. The 6-year molars are also instrumental in guiding the jaw even further in its growth process and shaping.

The second or permanent set of teeth, are called succedaneous, from the Latin word *succedere*, which means "to follow after." But this word is seldom used, and most people refer to the second set of teeth as the permanent or secondary teeth.

Permanent teeth usually erupt in the same order as the primary teeth. They will either come in by forcing the primary tooth out, or more commonly, in front or behind the baby tooth. In either case, eventually they move forward or backward into their proper place. Permanent teeth are traditionally more yellow than primary teeth, and have rough, jagged edges that wear down with age.

By the age of 16 most children will have all of their permanent teeth (with the exception of the wisdom teeth), so you should be able to count 28 teeth total, 14 on top and 14 on the bottom.

◆ Eruption Sequence ◆

Each child has an individual rhythm and pattern of acquiring teeth. There is no specific timetable because every child is unique. During the past 15 years, I have observed that approximately 70 percent of children experience a fairly routine pattern in their tooth eruption, whereas the other 30 percent experience a pattern that seems to have no rhyme or reason.

I recall one boy, whose first two teeth were his top central incisors. The next one to erupt was a top bicuspid or first molar. Another little girl acquired her bottom lateral incisors first. This created a very unique smile as she was missing her two front teeth.

Every child is different. I have met 3-year-olds who had only eight teeth, and 18-month-olds with 20 teeth. In some children, the 6 year molars start coming in as early as 4-and-a-half years, or as late as 8 years.

Here is what a traditional timetable might look like:

Lower primary teeth
6 months	= central incisors – cutting teeth
7 1/2 months	= lateral incisors
16 months	= cuspids or canines
12 months	= first molars or bicuspids – grinding and chewing teeth
20 months	= 2nd molars – grinding & chewing teeth

Upper primary teeth
7 months	= central incisors – cutting teeth
9 months	= lateral incisors
18 months	= cuspids or canines
14 months	= first molars or bicuspids – grinding and chewing teeth
24 months	= 2nd molars – grinding and chewing teeth

There are different theories as to how a sequence of eruption occurs. Some experts think that genetics are the guiding factor; others think jaw structure, cranial alignment or restrictions are influential; or that assimilation and processing of nutrients and minerals holds the key. Perhaps the timing is simply by chance.

Teeth buds are formed in utero and begin moving towards the gum line for their future eruption long before there is any visual evidence. A newborn infant is already involved in the teething process.

There are four levels of distinction within the teething process: mild, medium, intense and the teething rest period. The visual part of the teething process usually begins sometime between the sixth and eighth month with the eruption of the first tooth. The most common sequence of eruption starts with the two lower central incisors, and then the two upper central incisors. The lateral incisors follow these teeth at around 9 months. Between 12 and 14 months the first molars erupt, skipping a space and leaving room for the canines, which usually appear between 16 and 18 months. The second molars finally erupt between 18 and 30 months.

Once the 2-year molars have completed their eruption process, the child goes into a "teething rest period." This rest period will last until the first permanent teeth (6-year molars and/or the central incisors) start moving, which can begin anytime after 4-and-a-half years. The movement of these teeth can then precipitate some of the teething symptoms that the child experienced as an infant and toddler (i.e., ear or sinus infection, fever, diarrhea, irrational behavior, sleeplessness, fears, headaches, rashes, etc.) to reoccur.

A child will go through many changes during this teething rest period, both emotionally and physically, including the first real growth in height. Consequently, when the teeth start moving around again, anytime after the fourth birthday, a parent may not associate the recurrence of certain symptoms and behaviors with the earlier teething picture. Yet many parents will say to me, "What's wrong with Sarah? She is acting like she did when she was a baby."

The teething cycle will influence many aspects of the child between the ages of 5 and 14 years as the primary teeth fall out and the permanent ones come in. Some philosophers consider 6 and 7 years of age to be as important as the transition into puberty.[4]

The first few years (5 to 7 years) of this teething transition can be challenging for both child and parent, and will fall into the category of an "intense" teething period. Even if a child didn't have trouble with teething as an infant, acquiring 6-year molars may create some discomfort, behavior and emotional problems. It is during this time that many children are also diagnosed with attention deficit disorder or hyperactivity. There are many reasons why a child would display these behaviors. Teething is one of them. *(See chapter on "Natural Remedies for Teething Related Symptoms.")* The connection between teething and behavior is evident by simply observing the child.

If the child is on a fairly traditional timetable, the intensity of teething calms down between 7 and 8 years to a "medium" phase. Then, somewhere between 8 and 9 years, it will go to a "mild" phase, which only lasts until the bicuspids or premolars start erupting, moving back to a medium phase. When the 12-year molars start coming in, along with the exchange of many other teeth, it once again becomes an "intense" phase. Patience is a real virtue for a parent during this time.

Wisdom teeth, or third molars, are the last teeth to develop and appear. They are called "wisdom teeth" because they usually appear during a person's late teens or early twenties, which has been called the "age of wisdom." However, these teeth truly are unpredictable and can arrive anytime between the ages of 14 and 35 years. Some people never get wisdom teeth or will only get one or two of them because of a genetic disposition where they never form.

If the teenager's mouth has enough room, chances are the teeth will come in without any problems. *(See chapter on "Correcting Crooked Teeth.")* Unfortunately, a majority of the time this is not the case and the wisdom teeth will need to be extracted.

If there isn't enough room, several things can happen – teeth crowding will inhibit proper growth, causing an impaction, or incomplete development of the tooth; the tooth will come in at an angle and press on the molar next to it, causing pain to all teeth or damage to the neighboring tooth; or it will affect sinus passages or miscellaneous related nerves.

Once it has been established that extraction is the best course of action, you will be asked to sign a consent form acknowledging all of the possible complications related to the procedure. Dentist and oral surgeon George Maranon, D.D.S., says the most common problems that occur include pain of varying degrees, jaw swelling, bleeding and/or bruising. In rare cases, there may be more severe complications such as, an injury to the inferior alveolar nerve, an artery and/or vein or a jaw fracture. Maranon also cautions that these cases are rare and encourages patients to discuss any concerns about these outcomes with their surgeons on an individual basis. The main factors that put a patient at risk are the age at which the surgery takes place and the state of impaction – if it is superficial the percentage of risk is less, whereas if the roots are deep and close to a nerve, the risk is much higher.

Maranon says it is easier to extract wisdom teeth before they have completely formed, somewhere between the ages of 15-18 years. The best preventive measure you can take is to try and make room for the wisdom teeth when the child is younger with orthodontic procedures such as growth guidance, which offers the most expansive development for the jaw's fullest potential. Sometimes however, genetically the jaw is just too short to accommodate the teeth despite your best efforts. *(See chapter on "Correcting Crooked Teeth.")*

◆ Emotional, Spiritual & ◆ Physical Growth Patterns

Understanding the emotional, physical, and spiritual growth patterns of a child can give you more insight into the different levels of stress children endure.

A 2-year-old with the "terrible twos," a 5-year-old suddenly becomes irrational and out of control, or perhaps your 12-year-old is acting especially willful – take a deep breath, it may be related to the eruption of more teeth.

It takes approximately three years for a child to get her first set of teeth and 12 to 15 years for the completion of the exchange between these teeth and the full set of permanent teeth. True "teething" really begins at the age of 5. It is this second phase of teething that will influence your child's physical, emotional and behavior patterns for the next 15 years.

There are early childhood specialists who believe these behaviors are most specifically linked to particular developmental stages and would never consider the aspects of teething as a contributing factor. But my personal observations over the past 15 years have revealed that teething is an important component to this equation.

♦ Rudolf Steiner – An Austrian Philosopher ♦

Rudolf Steiner, an Austrian philosopher whose teachings form the basis of Waldorf Schools, realized these correlations and presented this information in his lectures and schools. He believed the oral stage was the first stage of the emotional development of human beings and states, "The first part of a child's life, up to the change of teeth, is spent with the unconscious assumption: the world is moral. The second period, from the change of teeth to adolescence, is spent with the unconscious assumption: the world is beautiful. And only with adolescence dawns the possibility of discovering: the world is true." The Waldorf schools reflect Steiner's philosophy and believe that a child is not ready to read, write or begin schooling until their teeth have started to transition or fall out.

The Encyclopedia Britannica describes Rudolf Steiner as the most universal genius of modern times. Others call him one of humanity's great spiritual teachers. As an Austrian philosopher, scientist and artist, he grew up with the clairvoyant certainty of a spiritual world. After schooling himself in modern science, he developed anthroposophy. Anthroposophy is a spiritual science described by Steiner as "a path of knowledge leading the spiritual in man, to the spiritual in the universe." His research into the developmental stages of our children opens a path of wisdom on many levels for a conscious parent's mind.

Steiner's philosophy of the spiritual aspects concerning a child's developmental stages is clearly defined in Bernard Lievegoed's book, *Phases of Childhood*. It is through his superbly written book, based on Steiner's philosophy, that I was able to better understand his ideas and pass them on to you. Any reference to Lievegoed in this chapter is merely his interpretation of the statements and thoughts of Steiner's philosophy.

♦ *A Child's Development:* ♦ *Physiological & Psychological*

The division of child's development from infancy to adulthood takes place in three seven-year cycles. This chapter primarily focuses on the first two phases and a portion of the third phase: Birth to 7 years, 7 to 14 years and 14 to 21 years. The first seven years of life can be divided into three categories: infancy, toddler and the period of transition towards school age.

Infancy: Birth-2 years

Babies double their birth weight in the first five months of life. An infant is completely dependent on its environment for everything at this time. It is very important that an infant sleeps, eats and has all of her needs met as she goes through these tremendous changes. Usually, the first tooth arrives between 5 and 6 months (but as we already know, there is no real timetable).

Over the next two years, the teething process will play a big role in all aspects of your child's life. A large percentage of children will acquire all 20 deciduous teeth during this period and their body weight will double again between 5 months and 2 years of age.

In addition to the physical growth and teething that take place during the first two years, an infant/toddler also goes through many other learning experiences such as: sensory development (i.e., visual, audio, olfactory and tactile); motor development (i.e., locomotion, sitting, crawling and creeping, standing and walking); language development and response capabilities.

A small child is a sensory organ in which desire and will are active. They are creatures of imitation and are extremely impressionable at a deep level reaching the most profound unconscious dimensions of the soul. It is these impressions that form a foundation for more conscious experiences later. A child is greatly influenced by their environment, which we as parents create for them during these first years of life.

◆ Transition From Infancy to Toddler Stage ◆

The transition from infancy to toddler is a wondrous accomplishment, especially when you consider that all higher mammals live their entire lives on a horizontal plane and never stand upright. Yet, as human beings, this is simply part of our evolution. The process normally begins in the second half of the first year, starting with the child's ability to roll over, sit up, crawl and then pull himself up.

Most children start walking in the second year of life, although there are many who start as early as 9 months. When a child starts to walk, it is considered the end of babyhood, and the beginning of toddlerhood. During this period the perceptive process has awakened and the child has conquered part of the outside world. This step also begins the first type of memory, and through rhythmic repetition, certain reflexes and habits are formed.

Speech follows shortly after this upright position has been achieved. Lievegoed writes, "When a child learns to speak, a spiritual order is laid down ... Language reflects the spiritual values, which are dominant in man at any given moment ... Learning to speak brings a breaking of the ties between the core of the self and the surrounding world, a process that only ends with puberty." In other words, thinking develops with and through speech.

Development of thought begins between the second and third year of life. This coincides with the eruption of the 2-year molars, which within itself can be an extremely difficult time physically. A child of so-called "normal development " will also develop a consciousness of self around this time.

This is also the beginning of the first negative stage, a period of obstinacy.

Many books describe this as the "terrible twos." I firmly believe that the "terrible twos" are directly related to the teething process with the eruption of the 2-year molars. Once these molars are in, the "terrible twos" soon become the "tender twos." Yes, you are still dealing with the psychological aspects of a 2-year-old, but without the physical discomfort of the incoming teeth. (I've noticed that girls tend to get their teeth earlier than boys.)

Depending on a child's teething schedule, there is usually a rest period between the ages of 3 and 4-and-a-half years. Even though there is no physical evidence of the teeth during this time, they will continue to silently move into position for their future eruption.

◆ 4-5 years ◆

Around the age of 4 years children start to see themselves as separate from the outside world, described as embarking on "creative imagination." This new phase stands in contrast to the outside world and can be changed according to the child's inner needs. A cushion is a car, and a closet is a house. Their imagination is now linked to reality. This is a time where fairy tales can awaken a child's spirit.

The feelings a child experiences at this age are at a level of the semiconscious dream state. It is at this age the child has their first growth of breadth (width).

At 5 years, children are deeply engulfed in imaginative play. They are continuously moving, absorbed by the rhythm and joy of their creation. Some may perceive this movement or restlessness as a form of hyperactivity. Usually it is between the age of 5 and 6 years that well-meaning school officials suggest prescription medications to calm and center a child. Sometimes tempers and moods can be extremely irrational during this period. Diet-related behavior should also be examined.

A child will also experience their first growth in height as the 6-year molars are preparing to erupt, presenting uncomfortable internal and external physical and emotional sensations. This can be an extremely volatile time and many of the old teething symptoms from infancy and toddlerhood reappear.

✦ 6-9 years ✦

The rhythmic process changes only slightly at the age of 6 years with the loss of the first milk tooth as the child enters the next stage of life. This is when the teething process truly begins. The eruption of the first 6-year molar usually takes place simultaneously with the loss of the first baby tooth, or shortly thereafter. Steiner believed it is at this point, and not before, that the structure of the soul is ready to start the learning process through schooling.

Goals are the next element added to the forces of creative play. This phase is a time of setting goals and striving for their achievement. The child gradually acquires an awareness of his own inability to achieve in reality things he sees in his imagination. This awareness creates a division between the child and the outside world. Now he needs assistance in his creative process, "Help me make a boat that will float or a paper airplane that will fly." This also leads to an infinite respect for the adult capable of participating with results and answers, a true figure of authority.

Seven to 14 years marks the second phase of development. The age between 7 and 9 years is considered the first metamorphosis of thinking. At the age of 7, the body goes through another structural change in the face, as the jaw grows further forward and the 6-year molars are either in the process of erupting or are already in.

Psychologically, the child moves from perception to concepts, which are real, yet unreal, a type of daydream. Words and stories are very important to a 7-year-old, for it is through language and words that the development of thinking is possible. This is when memory expands and becomes continuous and a child can learn to formulate conclusions to unanswered questions. Between the age of 2 and 8 years the body will also double its weight again.

◆ 9-12 years ◆

The next phase is from 9 to 12 years, when the child undergoes a transfor-
mation of feelings. This change takes place in the child's relation to the
outside world. Their protection of the imaginative world, which is externally projected, is lost. This can represent a sense of betrayal as their world is
now seen through different eyes. Suddenly, the child will have a fear of the
dark whereas a few months ago there was none. According to Steiner's
philosophy, these changes also bring shades of intolerance, indecision and
difficult mood swings, arising from satisfaction or dissatisfaction with the
world. Fortunately, a child's opposition to the outside world is still
expressed through words and feelings rather than actions. Criticism is also
awakened during this time, and there is a second growth in breadth.

This can be a very intense teething period. My daughter had nine teeth
coming in when she was 10 years old. She was extremely volatile in her
moods and behaviors. As adults, we can only imagine the physical pain or
strange sensations all of these changes can evoke.

If a child has not already been introduced to the wonders of nature by this
time, it can prove to be an excellent guiding tool for this phase. There is
usually a loss of respect for most authority figures and nature can provide
a whole new world, one that can be respected. Hero worship is also
awakened during this stage and if not properly guided, the child may reach
out for inappropriate idols, and inevitably meet disappointment.

◆ 12-14 years ◆

The stage of pubescence occurs between the ages of 12 and 14 years.
Another growth in height at 12 years adds new dimensions at a time when
a child begins to experience a total separation of her own personality from
the outside world. This propels their activities to be aimed at conquering
the outside world as a whole. For most kids, this is when the 12-year
molars are erupting along with several other teeth. Teething, coupled with
hormones and feelings of separation, can present a very stressful time
physically, emotionally and spiritually.

Some boys take on an aggressive, dominating behavior and want to partake in initiation games for the adventure, as well as to satisfy the urge to conquer. If this is not guided in a positive and constructive way, there can be severe consequences in society. They can also move into a highly physical achievement mode at this time, filled with excess energy and vitality. They have now acquired a realistic understanding for the situations that surround them.

Girls lean more towards forming groups, but also tend to go more inward at this age, becoming more mysterious. Usually their groups are small, three or four girls, sharing their innermost secrets with each other. The development of the will for some children can produce an aggression that is directed more towards their parents through bad tempers, depression, obstinacy and indecision. These behaviors are also symptomatic of the teething process. There is also another growth in height at this age, along with the development of breasts and for some, the onset of menstruation. Because of these extreme physical, hormonal and psychological changes, many girls become fatigued and require additional sleep.

For some young teens, this age can be very lonely. This is true for boys and girls. There is a strong sense of being different, separate and that no one understands them. If proper attention is given to children during this phase, their feelings of loneliness and being separate can be guided in a positive direction of self-empowerment.

Again, these behaviors are greatly influenced by the child's teething schedule. Since my daughter's teeth were on the early side, when she was in this age group, most of the time she was in the most wondrous of moods and extremely expressive. She was very present and wanted to participate in more social activities with me than ever before.

◆ Social Maturation ◆

Age 14 begins the third cycle of development and social maturation. Leivegoed describes the 14-year-old with three key thoughts: "Synthesis of thought; World-view; Sexual maturity." For the 16-year-old: "Synthesis of feeling; Religious inclination; Third growth in breadth." And the 18-year-old: "Synthesis of the will; Social responsibility; Preparing for a career; continuing to mature to manhood or womanhood."

During this period of social maturation, some late teething teens may still be working on getting their 12-year molars, while others prepare for the eruption of their wisdom teeth. Whatever the case, the teething process will continue to be a source of added stress influencing many aspects of a young adult.

◆ A Timeline On Teething - Chart ◆

Intensity of teething and physical symptoms

A. Intense = any combination, or one of the following symptoms – runny nose • nasal congestion, at times green or yellowish in color • sore throat • headache • vomiting • fever stomach ache • diarrhea • earache • sleeplessness • irritable coughs • teeth grinding • drooling • hyperactive • unable to concentrate or short attention span (similar behavior as ADD or ADHD).

B. Medium = fever • irritable • earache • runny nose • nasal congestion • cough • diarrhea • sleeplessness • drooling.

C. Mild = a mild version of any of the above symptoms.

Editor's Note: **It is important to thoroughly evaluate all symptoms for the possibility of a more serious health condition. Always consult your physician.**

(See chart on opposite page.)

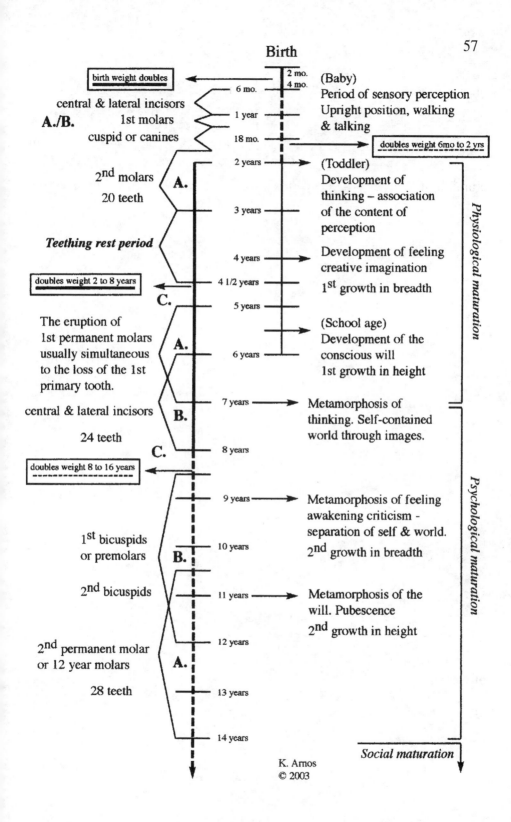

57

Birth

2 mo.
4 mo.

birth weight doubles

6 mo.

A./B. central & lateral incisors
1st molars
cuspid or canines

1 year

18 mo.

(Baby)
Period of sensory perception
Upright position, walking
& talking

doubles weight 6mo to 2 yrs

2 years

A. 2nd molars
20 teeth

3 years

(Toddler)
Development of
thinking – association
of the content of
perception

Teething rest period

4 years

Development of feeling
creative imagination

doubles weight 2 to 8 years

4 1/2 years

1st growth in breadth

C.

5 years

The eruption of
1st permanent molars
usually simultaneous
to the loss of the 1st
primary tooth.

A.

6 years

(School age)
Development of the
conscious will
1st growth in height

central & lateral incisors

7 years

B.

Metamorphosis of
thinking. Self-contained
world through images.

24 teeth

C.

8 years

doubles weight 8 to 16 years

9 years

Metamorphosis of feeling
awakening criticism -
separation of self & world.
2nd growth in breadth

1st bicuspids
or premolars

B.

10 years

2nd bicuspids

11 years

Metamorphosis of the
will. Pubescence
2nd growth in height

12 years

2nd permanent molar
or 12 year molars

A.

28 teeth

13 years

14 years

Physiological maturation

Psychological maturation

Social maturation

K. Amos
© 2003

"She brings you money…she has white wings and is little like my finger. She lives at the tooth fairy home in the sky. She takes her teeth to work and looks at them on her computer. She is pretty and loves me. I have lots of loose teeth and maybe they will come out at 6, 7 or 9." (Two weeks after this interview, Isabella lost her first tooth.)

Isabella - 5 years old

"I think the tooth fairy looks like a person with wings. The tooth fairy is one centimeter tall and is a girl. She feels like a pillow and looks like a fly. She gets all the teeth in the world by flying and does it when you are asleep. She does it because she is nice."

Michael - 8 years old

"The tooth fairy looks like a fly. It acts like a fly. It feels like a fly."

Randy - 5 years old

"The tooth fairy looks like a bird and flies. She is one foot long and feels soft. She lives in a castle. What she does is squashes under the pillow at midnight. That's what fairies do."

Abraham - 6 years old

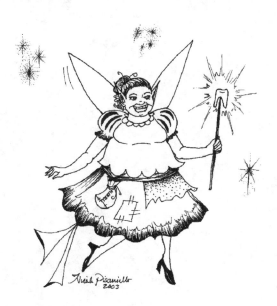

Chapter Three

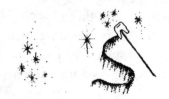

Breastfeeding – Bottle-feeding How They Affect Tooth & Jaw Development
Infant Formula • Thumb Sucking • Pacifiers

There was a time, long ago, when almost all newborn infants were breastfed. If a mother was unable to nurse her own baby she would find another woman with milk to help feed her infant. But over the years, the natural instincts of breastfeeding declined tremendously, reaching its lowest point ever in this country in 1971.[1]

In the late 90s, motherhood brought with it a renewed interest in breastfeeding. Today more than 60 percent of mothers nurse their babies.[2] Even though a minority of doctors are not up to date on current research, a majority of them are now better educated about the benefits of breastfeeding (nutritional, health, immunologic, cognitive, developmental, social, economic, and physiological).[3]

Whether or not to breastfeed is an important, individual decision; breastfeeding is not for everyone. For those who can and want to nurse their infants, the benefits can be tremendous. Many dentists and orthodontists agree that breastfeeding plays a big part in an infant's tooth and jaw

development. There are both physical and nutritional differences between a baby who is breastfed and one who is bottle-fed. This does not mean that bottle-fed babies won't have good teeth, but there are dental advantages to breastfeeding.

There are many reasons why a woman may not be able to nurse her infant: the child is adopted, the mother must return to work for economic or career reasons, physical abnormalities, immune problems, not enough milk and/or personal choice. The purpose of this chapter is to supply educational information on the benefits of breastfeeding, with regard to tooth and jaw development. It is in no way meant to judge or discourage parents who have made the decision to bottle-feed their infants.

♦ *Physiological Differences* ♦

Physiological differences exist between breastfed and bottle-fed infants. The choices a new mother makes may affect her baby's structural development.

The physiological aspects of breastfeeding are unique. The structure and consistency of breast tissue is nature's perfect source for creating proper teeth and jaw alignment and teaches the infant optimal swallowing patterns. When the breast is in the infant's mouth, it becomes completely flat, allowing the lips to almost meet. The breast is compressed on top of the tongue during the feeding, which encourages proper tongue movement and swallowing technique.

The entire process begins with the infant sucking and chewing hard with its mouth around the entire areola. The milk is extracted by squeezing the nipple with the tongue. The structure of a breast consists of an outer layer of fat and the glands that produce the milk. The milk is carried to the ducts in drops and moves towards the nipple where it comes out through many little holes. A mother's milk doesn't start flowing immediately. The infant stimulates the breast with its strong jaw muscles (considered to be three times stronger than an adult's), which cue the mother's body to release, or let down, the milk. The process takes a lot of work on the part of the baby.[4]

Once the milk is let down, the baby needs to keep working by advancing her lower jaw and chewing, to continue to draw drops of milk out of the breast. This action helps the jaw by strengthening the muscles and shaping the bones with a constant pulling motion. Marc Harmon, D.D.S., states, "I feel that the exercise of breastfeeding helps the jaw develop to its fullest potential, increasing the range of motion to the temporal bone and providing more room for better spacing of the teeth... In my practice, I've observed that bottle-fed babies seem to have a higher need for orthodontic treatment and/or teeth extractions due to a lack of space in the mouth."

Harmon also believes that the bonding time that goes along with feeding is very important – the womblike cradling, the touch, the eye to eye contact – "Love is the single most critical nutrient of all." If you do bottle-feed, he cautions, don't just prop the baby up with the bottle and walk away. It is important for both of you to honor this time together by holding him close to your body to experience the one-on-one bonding that takes place.

The physiological aspects of bottle-feeding present a different picture. Today there are various bottle nipples that try to replicate the shape of a woman's breast while nursing. When an infant drinks from a bottle, several things take place: The rubber nipple is thick and forces the lips to part; consequently, the jaw works differently and abnormal pressure is applied to the gums and, eventually, the teeth. The tongue's normal rhythm is disrupted by having to dance around the rubber nipple, where it is then allowed to push up against the teeth as it fills in the open spaces on both sides of the nipple. The milk flows more easily from the nipple of a bottle in comparison to a woman's breast, which forces the infant to use his tongue to control the flow and prevent choking. This unnatural feeding pattern can create what is known as "tongue thrusting."

Harmon adds, "Tongue thrusting refers to the placement of the tongue between the teeth, and contributes to abnormal bite relationships, mouth development and appearance." He continues, "The functional difference between a normal swallow and a thrusting swallow can result in a narrow face producing a high palate, narrow arch, reduced sinus spaces, as well as possible effects to the pineal gland and cerebral development. This can occur when there is a lack of tongue stimulation to the maxillary arch during development."[5]

Another drawback to most bottle nipples is that they require little effort from an infant's jaw muscles. According to Marvin S. Eiger, M.D. and Sally Wendkos Olds, authors of *The Complete Book of Breastfeeding*, it is this lack of exercise in a bottle-fed baby that can result in what is known as a "lazy jaw."[6]

Donald Getz, D.O., an optometrist specializing in visual development, advises parents to remember to switch sides (left, right) when bottle-feeding to encourage visual wellness in both eyes. Getz believes that if you continuously feed your baby in the same position, her eyes will not be equally exercised. "This child is likely to have an eye coordination problem which could lead to academic difficulties when she goes to school." And Arnold Gesell, M.D., of the Gesell Institute of Child Development, states, "Vision is the dominant process in child development."[7]

If you choose to bottle-feed there are steps you can take to help promote healthy jaw and tooth development. First, use a nipple that most resembles a mother's nipple when it is in the mouth of the infant. Second, look for a nipple with a smaller hole to encourage the child to work harder and exercise the jaw muscles as much as possible. By using a nipple with a smaller hole, the tongue won't be used as frequently to regulate the flow of milk, which will help encourage healthier tongue patterns. (The Nuk nipple is the only one I would recommend at this time; 1-800-4-Gerber.)

◆ *Nutritional Differences* ◆

According to the American Academy of Pediatrics, "Breastfeeding is the ideal method of feeding and nurturing infants." It recognizes breastfeeding as a primary source for achieving optimal infant and child health, growth and development.[8] The AAP also states, "Epidemiologic research in the United States, Canada, Europe and other developed countries shows that human milk and breastfeeding of infants significantly decreases the incidence and/or severity of diarrhea, lower respiratory infections, otitis media, bacteremia, bacterial meningitis, botulism, urinary tract infections and more."[9]

As the late Benjamin Spock once said, "Breast milk is best for babies." Breast milk is specifically made for a baby's unique needs. It has an intricate and reliable composition; the beginning of the feeding or fore milk, offers a high-protein milk, whereas the end or hind milk is high-fat, which gives the infant a sense of fullness.[10]

♦ Mother's Milk ♦

There are three stages of breast milk: *colostrum* – the first secretion from the breast after childbirth, which comes 24 to 48 hours after birth and lasts from four to five days; *transitional milk* - a mixture of colostrum and mature milk, which lasts approximately two weeks; and mature milk - the complete milk, also known as true milk.[11]

♦ Colostrum ♦

One of the most important immune-building properties of breast milk comes from colostrum. Colostrum is the pre-milk fluid produced from the mother's mammary glands during the first 24 to 48 hours after birth. Humans are born with immature immune systems. While the immune systems of babies develop, their bodies are supported by the nutrients in colostrum.

The composition of colostrum is different from mature milk. Colostrum is easier to digest, and contains more nutrients such as proteins, minerals, vitamins, complex carbohydrates and more. Studies show that colostrum contains powerful immune factors such as immunoglobulins, lactoferrin, cytokines, interferon and PRP (Polyproline-Rick-Peptides.)[12]

According to health researcher and writer Beth Ley, "The colostrum provided in breast milk contains all the needed immune factors which are of great significance as the newborn's own system develops." Among these factors are antibodies against infections such as *E. coli*, salmonella, cholera, pneumonia, pertussis, diphtheria, strep and candida.[13]

Besides helping to protect against infection, colostrum promotes growth, advances the maturity of the stomach and digestive tract, signals the brain to regulate digestion, and offers a unique combination of high-energy nutrients that ensure proper development of the brain and nervous system. In addition, it contains enzyme inhibitors, which protect it from destruction in the gastrointestinal tract. According to physician and author Zoltan

Rona, M.D., "It is estimated that colostrum triggers at least 50 processes in the newborn."[14]

♦ *Transitional Milk* ♦

Human milk contains 100 ingredients that are not found in cow's milk, and changes in composition continuously as the baby grows. In addition to the three initial stages of milk development over the first month, the human body continues to regulate its chemistry. The components change during a single feeding, over a day, a month, even over years. Mother's milk produces different quantities of certain constituents at different times or phases to support the different nutritional needs of the developing child. A 6-week-old infant has different needs than a 6-month- or a 2-year-old toddler (i.e., the milk produced for a premature infant will be different from the milk produced for a child who is being weaned). Changes in the weather also affect the composition: a hot summer day will produce milk with more water in it to properly hydrate a more frequently nursing child without giving her too many vitamins.

Unfortunately, infant formula does not possess these natural intuitive capabilities. So if a baby is drinking more formula to quench his thirst during the summer he may be receiving too much supplementation, which can put a strain on immature organs.[15]

Breast milk also contains docosahexaenoic acid, or DHA, an essential fatty acid important for proper development. During the last half of pregnancy, the fetus holds on to more of this fat than other fats in the mother's bloodstream. In turn, a breastfeeding infant will receive appropriate amounts of DHA, supplied by the mom, whereas a baby that is formula fed will not.[16]

One of the primary nutritional differences between breast-fed and formula-fed babies is the amount of proteins. Cow's milk contains approximately two times as much protein as human milk, supplying the infant with more protein than is needed or can be absorbed, consequently putting more stress on the baby's elimination processes. This is one of the reasons formula-fed babies tend to be heavier in weight and have firmer stools. Breast-fed babies absorb and use 100 percent of the protein in breast milk, which also contains an enzyme to aid in its own digestion.[17]

Another benefit of mother's milk is that it can make specific antibodies to bacteria or viruses. These immunologic constituents include: macrophages, polymorpho-nuclear leukocytes, B- & T-lymphocytes, immunoglobulins, bifidous factor, lysozyme, lactoferrin and lactoperoxidase.[18] According to Eiger and Olds, "Women develop specific antibodies against bacteria and viruses in their own lungs and intestines, which also appear in their breast milk." This provides a child with optimal immunological benefits. The authors also state that, depending upon what the mother eats, the baby will become more familiar with varied tastes and smells that come through the breast milk.[19]

Considering the nutritional differences between breast milk and formula, it is clear that breast milk supplies the infant with the optimal nutrition for the development and growth of healthy bones and teeth.

◆ *Infant Formula* ◆

In most cases, children who are bottle-fed grow and develop normally and are quite healthy. The information you are about to read is not meant to scare you, but to educate you.

In the past few decades, there have been some problems with the manufacturing of infant formula, which was first brought to public awareness in 1978 when Syntex, a California-based company, accidentally left chloride out of its two infant formulas: Neo-Mull and Cho-free. According to Maureen Minchin, author of *Food for Thought, A Parent's Guide to Food Intolerance*, babies suffered a wide range of symptoms as a result of an abnormally high alkali content in their blood. The consequences included developmental delays, convulsions, failure to thrive, diarrhea, constipation, kidney defects and more.

Several other incidents of record include: salmonella bacteria found in an Australian manufactured formula, causing widespread illness; in 1978, a formula designed for premature babies contained indigestible curds formed by protein, which caused bowel obstructions; in 1980 Soy-a-lac and I-soy-a-lac were recalled as a result of too much vitamin D, which produced side effects such as kidney damage and convulsions.[20] In today's society, with the mass production of foods and other products, accidents are bound to happen.

The Syntex incident in 1980 led Congress to pass the "Infant Formula Act," which mandates that the Food and Drug Administration (FDA) ensure that formulas contain all the nutrients that babies need. But, what nutrients do infants need? Technology can only attempt to understand the intricacy of this formulation and try to replicate it to the best of their manufacturing ability.

Another of Minchin's concerns is that not all preparation mishaps of infant formula are publicized. For instance, deficiencies of essential fatty acids can result in skin, eye and gut disorders, and failure to thrive. Or if there is an excess of iron in the formula it can cause gastrointestinal bleeding, anemia and immunological disorders. Some formulas come in a can and may also pose the risk of lead or aluminum exposure to an infant.[21]

Moves to improve infant formula continue. Some companies now offer formulas for different developmental stages, which is a start towards a more efficient product. But still, some of the ingredients in infant and stage formulas are questionable. One Ohio-based company, Nature's One, Inc., has come out with an organic formula, Baby's Only Organic pediatric formula. Nature's One offers both a dairy or soy-based formula. The dairy formula is made with organic milk, free of bovine growth hormones, antibiotics and steroids. The soy formula is made using a patent-pending process that naturally breaks down two sugars, raffinoise and stachyoise, for easy digestion. Some baby formula manufacturers use a soy protein isolation process that chemically strips the soybean of many of its naturally occurring benefits. Nature's One also uses certified organic oils (i.e., soybean, high oleic sunflower and coconut oils), and sweetens their formula with organic brown rice syrup, rather than the traditional corn syrup. Corn syrup is the cheapest source of carbohydrate used in most infant formulas and is most likely made from genetically altered corn. Nature's One formulas also contain essential fatty acids, taurine and selenium, all of which are present in breast milk, but lacking in cow and soy milk.

Nature's One recommends consulting a health practitioner to establish appropriate proportions of their formula for infants less than 12 months of age. This is important advice when choosing any formula to ensure there are no food allergies or developmental issues that might require a specialty formula. The makers of Nature's One acknowledge there is nothing better for an infant than breast milk, but understand that circumstances sometimes necessitate the use of formula. It is nice to know there is a natural formula available to better meet this need.

Susan Roberts, Ph.D., Melvin Heyman, M.D., and Lisa Tracy, authors of *Feeding Your Child for Lifelong Health*, describe two essential fatty acids infants need – linoleic acid (LA) and alpha-linolenic acid (ALA). Both are used to synthesize new brain tissue. These two fatty acids make two other fatty acids – arachidonic acid and docosahexaenoic acid (DHA).[22] According to current science, DHA is a key ingredient still missing in most manufactured infant formula. This omega-3 fatty acid is found in fish oils and is one of the most prevalent fats in the human brain and the retina of the eye, making it an important factor in brain and eye development.[23]

In the book *Superimmunity* for Kids, Leo Galland, M.D., and Dian Dincin Buchman, Ph.D., explain that appropriate amounts of DHA during the first six months of life are critical for an infant's proper development. The best vegetable source of omega-3 ALA is flaxseed oil. The body uses this omega-3 EFA, through a conversion process, to manufacture DHA and EPA. It has a mild taste and is more palatable than fish oil. It should never have a rancid or bitter taste. If it does, it is spoiled and should be thrown away immediately. It can be added easily to an infant's formula. The authors suggest supplementation of up to one teaspoon a day divided into three feedings, added to room temperature formula.

Another vegetable source of omega-3 EFA is Perrila oil, a new product, which is a member of the mint family. Perrila oil is one of the richest sources of omega-3 EFA, giving it a slight edge over flaxseed oil on surviving the conversion process in making DHA and EPA. (It is important to note that hemophiliacs should use caution in the use of EFA in general, due to its blood thinning properties. Also those using mega doses of EFA's for therapeutic purposes should stop intake before surgical procedures. Always consult a medical doctor for any related questions.)

Galland and Dincin Buchman also suggest that gamma linolenic acid (GLA), found in evening primrose and black currant oil, can also be deficient in formula and may be supplemented topically by puncturing the capsule of oil and rubbing it into the skin of the infant. The oil is absorbed directly into the system through the skin. Always check with a nutritionist or knowledgeable person in this area as to what an appropriate source and ratio of EFA would be best for your child.[24]

Roberts, Heyman and Tracy also point out, "One recent study showed better problem solving ability at 10 months in babies whose formulas had been supplemented with just 1 to 1.5 grams per day of DHA, compared to babies fed with standard formula." And, "A recent study of teenagers born at full term and breast-fed for even a few weeks showed higher IQ, better school grades and only half the risk of leaving school early compared to teenagers fed formula after birth."[25]

Regardless of efforts to produce a precise infant formula, if it is made from a powdered mix, it has the potential of being inexact. Minchin feels, "If the scoop is pressed too hard, or not firmly enough, the results and changes in composition can be significant. For instance, too much of one component and not enough of another." She also cautions, "Formula feeding is based upon our limited knowledge of the components of human milk, with extra added for safety." So if you are using powdered infant formula, be sure to shake the can or package well before measuring and preparing each serving.

For currant information on infant formula recalls, go to http://safetyalerts.com/rcls/category/child.htm.

♦ Bottlemouth Syndrome ♦
Breastfeeding VS. Bottle-feeding to Sleep

Another debate among dentists is feeding an infant to sleep. The discussion begins with the eruption of the first tooth and those that follow. Once a tooth erupts, the health of the enamel and structure can be jeopardized if caution is not exercised. Depending on the overall genetics and nutritional foundation of the tooth, the prevention of decay is now an important concern.

The differences between bottle-feeding and breastfeeding an infant or child to sleep play an important role in the health of teeth. Breastfeeding triggers an automatic swallowing reflex, which clears the infant's mouth of milk, helping to prevent the milk from pooling or collecting in the mouth around the teeth.

If you bottle-feed your infant to sleep always be sure that all the liquid is swallowed and not left to pool in the mouth. To maintain an empty mouth after eating, gently rock the infant to trigger a swallowing response. Holding infants while feeding also gives them strong emotional support.

The real danger of bottle-feeding comes when a parent is tempted to give a crying child a bottle in the crib at night. In most cases, the nipple will continue to drip in the mouth even after the baby has fallen asleep, allowing the liquid to accumulate in the mouth and bathe the teeth for long periods. The enriched carbohydrates and strong acids from the formula will remain in contact with the teeth all night, resulting in what is called "bottlemouth syndrome."[26] *(See chapter on "Cavities and Decay.")*

• Thumb Sucking •

The sucking instinct is one of first natural instincts, often seen immediately after birth as a newborn is put to the breast or bottle and starts sucking. Ultrasound technology has now confirmed that thumb sucking actually begins in utero.

Rosemarie Van Norman, author of *Helping the Thumb Sucking Child* and a certified myologist (the study of oral-facial muscle function and its relationship to dental and speech development), states, "Sucking fixations and oral fixations in infants provide stimulation that is essential for the development of the central nervous systems. These are normal behaviors that teach babies to discern things such as temperature, texture, color, shape, size and proximity."[27]

Babies suck their thumbs, hands and fingers or use a pacifier for several reasons: to extend pleasure after feeding; the pressure on the gum feels good to a teething child; the child has a strong sucking urge that needs to be satisfied; to calm and/or center itself; to release emotional stress, anger or frustration; or a combination of the above.

It is said that 75 to 95 percent of infants in western cultures take part in thumb or finger sucking or use a pacifier. The habits are referred to as non-nutritive sucking, the action of sucking for purposes other than obtaining food or nutrition.[28] In 1976, the *Journal of Dentistry of Children* published a study that reported 19 percent of U.S. children continued thumb sucking past the age of 5. And, more recently a 1994 study found the percentage to be even higher. Twenty-six percent of children between the ages of 6 and 9 continued to suck their thumbs.[29] Even Sigmund Freud discusses the merits of what he calls "pleasure sucking" in his 1912 lecture, "General Introduction to Psychoanalysis."[30]

In Van Norman's work with children, she found that out of 723 kids, 34 percent began habitual sucking behavior on a pacifier. She states, "When infants who had become used to a pacifier developed the motor skills to bring their thumbs to their mouths at will, they would suck their thumbs whenever the pacifier wasn't available." Children may also start thumb sucking when a parent is trying to wean them of their pacifier, and find their thumbs as a substitute.[31]

Thumb sucking can affect the direction of growth of the facial structures. It encourages a downward growth pattern. Fortunately, because the bones are soft, pliable and still growing until approximately 12 years old, there are successful correctional techniques that can remedy malocclusion caused by thumb sucking. *(See chapter on "Correcting Crooked Teeth.")*

Pressure applied during thumb sucking influences the position of teeth and bones in the upper and lower dental arches. Prolonged sucking can cause many problems: structural changes to developing jaw bones and teeth; speech impediments; difficulties with social relationships, school work, and self-esteem; and, in rare cases, the habit can affect the formation of the thumb or fingers and/or knuckle bones.[32] The degree of damage depends on the severity of the habit and overall genetics.

In her book, Van Norman describes the physiological aspects of the pleasure involved with the act of sucking. The brain has the ability to manufacture its own mood-altering chemicals and "has billions of nerve cells that communicate with one another through neurotransmission – the sending of nerve impulses from one part of the body to another ... Neurotransmission stimulates the brain to produce certain chemicals and thus controls all emotions, perceptions, and bodily functions." Thumb sucking stimulates the brain to produce these chemicals.[33]

Van Norman also states, "As the child sucks, the brain produces chemicals called enkephalins and related compounds called endorphins, which decrease neurotransmission. Decreased neurotransmission produces a calming, relaxing sensation. Thumb-sucking causes this type of neuro-transmission." These endorphins reduce pain and offer a tranquilizing effect to an infant's or child's emotions and physical body.[34]

Harmon believes that the physical deformities resulting from thumb sucking are potentially not as serious as the emotional problems that can develop when a child is constantly reminded that she is doing something wrong. As for the physical repercussions, he states, "The effects and treat-ment of thumb sucking are not easily discussed from a general point of view. The adverse effects will be unique and specific to the individual and will depend on the intensity and strength of the muscle's actions and vacuum forces, among other considerations."[35]

Harmon describes one of his patients in her 30s who still sucks her thumb – her two front teeth have been bonded together from the rear to keep them from opening a midline space. She still shows no obvious problems with her mouth or face as a result. However, he has seen 4-year-olds who are already exhibiting facial and dental deformities as a result of thumb suck-ing. "Fortunately, in my office, with the use of cranial adjustments and Crozat therapy I have been able to correct most problems caused by thumb sucking habits."[36]

To better understand the dynamics of thumb sucking, try sucking your own thumb. What happens is a shift in the upper part of your jaw, a rotation forward with an upper thrust, and the teeth hit against the knucklebone of the thumb.

Taking the process and the physical awareness you have just experienced, imagine what consequences a child's bones may endure. Their bones are much softer and more malleable than an adult's. The thrust of the thumb into the arch forces the front teeth to be pushed forward, which causes a narrowing of the jaw. This can lead to problems with jaw development, spacing and positioning of the teeth. When a child is repeating this process on a daily basis, in some cases for years, changes are bound to occur.

◆ *Pacifiers* ◆

A pacifier can be an important comforting tool. Unfortunately, this tool can influence the developing facial structures of your infant or child, so it is important to use one that meets appropriate orthodontic criteria such as the Nuk Orthodontic Pacifier. Gerber offers the pacifier in two different materials: latex and silicon. A spokesperson for the company states, "We now offer the silicon material because some children have an allergy to latex." The latex pacifier comes in three different sizes, 0-6 months, 6-18 months and 18 months and up. The silicon only comes in two sizes, 0-6 months and 6-18 months.

Whatever pacifier you buy, be sure it is made of nontoxic, flexible material and has a strong one-piece construction. The mouth guard should not be removable from the nipple. Never attach a pacifier with a cord or string around a baby's neck. This is a hazard and many children have died of strangulation. Examine the pacifier frequently for pieces that may be wearing or that can come apart to ensure its durability and safety. Be sure to replace it accordingly.

"I like the tooth fairies – there is more than one tooth fairy, because they take your tooth and give you money. It's so exciting I have a wiggly tooth! I think they come in the night and you hide your tooth behind your pillow and they get it and then they leave you money. I think about two dollar bills, maybe, and a quarter…I don't know. Once they give it, then we'll know. They are small and they have little wings – pink wings that you can see through."

Cole – 5 years old

"I remember as a young girl waiting with my mother for a streetcar in downtown San Francisco, where I would see the ferry building. I thought that was where the tooth fairy lived. I could imagine her buzzing in and out of the clock tower."

Helen – Mother of three

"I had my first loose tooth and it was bothering me. My dad tried to pull it out with pliers. He put a paper towel over it and tried to pull it with the pliers – it didn't work. Later that day, my mom tried again with her hand and a paper towel, then it came out. I sewed a tooth fairy doll and it has a pocket on the front to put my tooth in. Then I put it under my pillow. The tooth fairy came and took the tooth, but I didn't see her. She left me a butterfly net – but you can't use it to catch fairies. She has white wings almost like a heart but you can't see her body, it is see-through. She lives at the bottom of the stream with the other fairies where she changes the teeth into crystals."

Gal – 6 years old

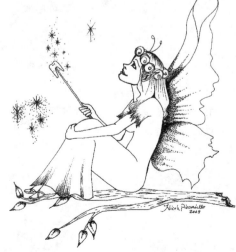

Chapter Four

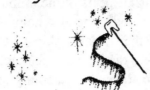

Natural Remedies for Teething-Related Symptoms

Behavioral & Emotional Reactions
Fever • Nose, Ears & Throat • Headaches • Croup
Coughs • Vomiting • Digestive Upset • Diaper Rash
Sleeplessness • Teeth Grinding and more

• Physical, Emotional & Behavioral Symptoms •

This chapter is based on my personal observations as a parent and as a natural healing consultant over the past 15 years. Once I realized there was a direct correlation between Danielle acquiring a new tooth, her behavior and physical symptoms, I began observing other children, eventually, witnessing the same relationships.

I repeatedly saw symptoms of physical illness, emotional and behavior problems specific to certain age groups occurring simultaneously with the eruption of teeth. These symptoms include fever, irritability, drooling, headaches, diarrhea, vomiting, diaper rash, sleeplessness, nightmares, stomachaches, teeth grinding, fatigue, fears, anxiety, depression, low self-esteem, ear and/or throat problems, sinus congestion, runny nose, cough, out-of-control behavior (categorized in young children as tantrums and in older ones as psychosis), and attention deficit disorder (ADD) or attention deficit hyperactivity disorder (ADHD.)

I think it is important to share this information and offer parents alternatives in working with their children's special needs during the teething process. It is our responsibility as parents to become more educated and familiar with the nutritional aspects of the immune system and the physiological mechanics of the body, thereby helping us to better understand different symptoms and their relationship to the body's functions. This knowledge will enable us to distinguish accurately, with caution, the difference between a symptom related to teething and a more serious health problem.

There are many professionals who don't agree with my theories regarding this connection between teeth and physical, emotional, and behavioral symptoms, but there are many parents that do, or who are open to exploring the idea. The following sections will discuss the symptoms most prominent in teething children from birth to adolescence and offer healthy solutions.

◆ *Fever* ◆

There are many reasons for a child to experience a fever – influenza, viral or bacterial infections, meningitis, appendicitis, roseola, chicken pox, cold, sinus infection, teething, etc. All possibilities need to be examined in the assessment of a situation before an educated decision can be made in regard to the treatment of a fever.

A fever is the body's defense mechanism in response to an infection or imbalance. Its purpose is to help defend the body against infections by increasing the production of white blood cells to fight viruses, bacteria or other harmful invaders. If the child is experiencing a temperature, it is a time to be observant and to make sure he is comfortable. According to pediatrician Kenneth Stoller, M.D., it isn't necessarily how high the fever is, within reason, but rather the child's response or behavior that will give you more insight into the severity of the situation. If, for instance, the temperature is 103°F and the child is actively playing, Stoller wouldn't be as concerned as if the fever is 101°F and the child is lethargic, uncomfortable or wants to sleep all day. He feels that the second behavior would be of more concern.[1]

The more you become familiar with your child's health patterns, the better you will be at recognizing a symptom associated with the teething process. Teething actually begins at birth. The teeth start pushing through gum tissue long before there are any visible signs of a tooth. As this process takes place, a child may experience a fever. Stoller feels the reason a fever occurs during this time is that as gum tissue is torn or destroyed by a moving tooth – an inflammatory response kicks in and chemical messengers are released into the bloodstream. This action signals the brain to turn up the thermostat. Depending on the amount and rate of tissue destruction in the individual, some children are affected and others are not. This was documented in a study at Tel Aviv University in February 1992, showing teething-related fevers starting up to 20 days prior to a tooth's eruption.[2]

Pay close attention to a fever that rises quickly, as it has a potential for producing seizures. If the child is experiencing extreme lethargy, stiffness of the neck or body, seizures, vomiting or labored breathing, get medical assistance immediately.

Self-help:

If a child does experience a fever related to teething, there are measures you can take to help support the immune system and still maintain a safe environment for the fever to do its job. A tepid bath with Epsom salts and lavender essential oil will help reduce a fever naturally. The appropriate homeopathic remedy will also be of assistance.

If the fever is above 102°F and the child is uncomfortable, an acetaminophen such as Tylenol, Tempra or other over-the-counter drug can be administered. Never give more than the recommended dosage for a child's size and body weight, as an excess of this drug can cause liver damage.[3] Never give aspirin to a child with a fever. It has been linked to Reye's syndrome, a progressive liver disease that can be fatal.

The most common homeopathic remedies to help relieve a fever associated with teething are:

Aconitum napellus – Sudden onset of fever; the child is fearful, restless, usually thirsty and pale; symptoms may come on after exposure to cold wind.

Belladonna – Sudden onset with throbbing pain; flushed hot face; the child may be delirious with little thirst.

Chamomilla – The child is irritable and continuously moaning for what he cannot have; one red cheek; easily angered; gas or diarrhea; extremely thirsty, wants to nurse continuously; not much appetite.

Ferrum phosphoricum - A slower onset, with no other symptoms.

Pulsatilla - The child is sad, weepy and wants to be cared for; very little thirst.

♦ *Drooling/Excessive Saliva* ♦

One of the symptoms associated with teething is drooling, which can be excessive at times. A child often experiences a constant flow of saliva long before a tooth actually erupts. When a tooth is pushing through gum tissue, the salivary glands produce extra saliva to keep the gum moist as the tooth breaks through the tissue.

The excess accumulation of saliva in the mouth can precipitate a cough, which becomes worse at night when lying down. The saliva pools in the mouth and drips down the back of the throat and into the chest. A teething cough can be persistent, sometimes lasting for weeks at a time. This cough is usually not helped by antibiotic treatment. This extra saliva production may occur periodically during any phase of the teething process.

Self-help:
The most common homeopathic remedies to help relieve drooling associated with teething are:

Mercurius vivus – There is constant drooling with redness of the gums, sometimes with little ulcers on the tongue and mouth.

Kreosote – The gums are protruding and the saliva is dark and watery.

◆ *Nose, Ears &' Throat* ◆

◆ *Nose* ◆

The most common reasons children experience a runny or stuffy nose are food allergies: dairy, chocolate, wheat, sugar, etc.; or environmental allergies, such as hay fever, pets, grass, flowers, bedding, stuffed animals, exposure to toxic elements, etc., a head cold or teething.

For many infants and toddlers, a runny nose is very common during the first 2-and-a-half years of life. The nose, ears and throat are all interconnected with the gums and teeth. Usually, the tearing of the gum tissue or eruption of a tooth will precipitate a clear discharge from the nose.[4] What I hear most often from a parent is, "It seems like my child is continuously sick. Her nose runs all the time."

Some children experience the opposite effect – a stuffy nose that can lead to a sinus infection. The nasal discharge starts out clear, but after a few days becomes cloudy, yellow or even green in color. This condition is usually more extreme and generally happens during the eruption of the 2-, 6-, and 12-year molars.

Self-help:
Both of these conditions can cause nasal passages to be raw or inflamed on the inside or outside of the nose. A nasal spray can help soothe and reduce inflammation to swollen membranes and heal rawness. A nasal wash can be prepared at home by mixing one-quart of warm water with a teaspoon of table or sea salt. Place a few drops in each nostril two times a day. There are also several natural nasal spray formulas available at health food stores or select local pharmacies. *(See resources in back of book.)*

A warm washcloth compress placed over the sinus area (be careful not to make it too hot) will help loosen a stuffed sinus passage. *(See resources in back of book – Eco Groovy.)* To make an inhalation treatment using essential oils consider the following scents: lavender, tea tree, eucalyptus, rosemary or chamomile (Roman or German). Add a few drops of the essential oil to slow running hot water in the bathroom sink. Have your child breath the vapors for up to 10 minutes if necessary. You can make a tent with a towel, and have the child close his eyes and mouth and breathe in the vapor. Be sure the steam is cool enough not to burn the face. An alternative, is the use of an aromatherapy vaporizer or diffuser – a waterless vaporizer is best because it won't encourage mold or bacteria growth. You can, however, add a few drops of essential oils to a traditional humidifier or vaporizer with similar results.

Encourage your child to drink as much water and/or decaffeinated herbal tea as possible. Avoid dairy products and fruit juices, especially orange juice, which contributes to excess mucus production.

◆ *Ears* ◆

Ear infections and the inflammation of the eustachian tube may also be related to the teething process. There are two classifications of ear infections – chronic or acute. A chronic condition is one that continues to recur or is long-standing. An acute condition is usually expressed through a sudden, intense pain. It is not uncommon for a child who suffers from chronic otitis media (middle ear condition) to also suffer from acute episodes.

During the teething process, especially when molars are moving into place or erupting, the eustachian tube may become inflamed. One of the functions of the tube is to drain excess fluid away from the eardrum. If the child is experiencing nasal congestion and the eustachian tube is not draining properly, the fluid can back up into the ear. Unfortunately, this stagnant fluid becomes an encouraging host for bacteria to grow and creates pressure on both sides of the eardrum, causing pain.[5]

You don't need to have nasal congestion to experience ear pain. Acute ear pain can come on suddenly without any previous cold symptoms. An infection can produce a variety of different symptoms – throbbing, a dull ache, dizziness, sharp stabbing pain, diminished hearing, etc.

There are different types of ear infections. The eardrum in a normal state is pearly-gray, shiny and somewhat transparent. It is this transparency that allows us to see if there is fluid or pus behind the eardrum. If there is fluid in the ear, there will be a visible fluid line that moves as the head is tilted from front to back (similar to a container filled with liquid, being tilted from side to side). There are three different fluids found in the ear. The most common fluid is serous, thin and watery, which usually does not contain harmful bacteria; the others are mucoid, which is sticky and thick, and purulent, a fluid with pus. The purulent fluid is the type that often contains harmful bacteria.[6]

Some children never show signs of an acute earache or infection, but every time they go to the doctor for a checkup, they are diagnosed with another ear infection. The diagnosis is usually made when the inner ear is red, inflamed or bulging. This condition is often not the result of a bacterial infection but rather instigated by a food or environmental allergy, or teething. Unfortunately, this is the point when antibiotics are usually prescribed. Antibiotics are only beneficial if the ear infection is of a bacterial nature, which it usually is not. In some cases, antibiotics will temporarily produce signs of improvement, but once the child is off them, the symptoms will return. One Swedish study showed recurrences were 40 percent more likely after treatment with antibiotics, and that ear infections cleared up respectively in the same amount of time with or without antibiotics.[7]

Many children become prisoners to the antibiotic merry-go-round – on repeated courses of antibiotics for endless bouts of ear or sinus infections. The cycle can last for months or even years. I have met hundreds of parents who have even put their kids on prophylactic antibiotic maintenance for chronic ear infections. My experience has taught me that if antibiotics are not working, there is usually another *causative factor* involved.

Here's how the antibiotic cycle works. A child is diagnosed with an ear infection, characterized by either acute pain or an otoscope examination. An antibiotic is prescribed, which not only kills invading bacteria but also kills the beneficial bacteria in the intestinal tract. These beneficial bacteria help control the delicate balance of intestinal yeast. When the good bacteria are destroyed, the yeast has a chance to multiply and become systemic in the body. One of the many symptoms of too much yeast in the system is a craving for sugar. Once this happens, the child becomes allergic to different foods and environmental sources. These allergic responses then express in a weakened immune system and show up as repeated ear infections (not necessarily bacterial), skin rashes, behavioral problems, yeast infections, thrush, etc.[8]

Self-help:

The best way to break the cycle and get off the antibiotic merry-go-round is through nutritional education. First, explore natural options in treating ear infections, i.e., homeopathy, herbs and chiropractic structural alignments. Arrest the yeast and start rebalancing the intestinal tract with beneficial bacteria. For infants to 7 years, use a non-dairy bifidus culture. For 7 years and older, a non-dairy acidophilous culture is most appropriate. Other supplements that can assist in the rebalancing process include, essential fatty acids, calcium, magnesium, zinc, vitamins A, C, B complex, echinacea, adrenal support and, of course, healthy eating habits. Children who follow this regimen tend to regain good health quickly.

The three main herbs used in eardrop formulations for the relief of ear pain are: garlic - used as a bacteria-fighting agent; mullein: used to break up congestion; and St. John's wort (hypericum): used to help relieve nerve pain. These herbs are usually combined with an olive oil, if possible, slightly warmed and placed in the ear a few drops at a time (nap or bedtime is best.) *(See resources in back of book.) Important note:* Never put an oil or tincture in an ear that is draining fluid.

Another herb, which is helpful for ear pain associated with teething, is plantago major. Simply place a few drops of the mother tincture directly into the ear. Colloidal silver can also be placed directly in the ear, 2-3 drops three times a day to help fight infection. Other effective ingredients include, grapefruit seed extract and Tea Tree oil. The flower essence *Rescue Remedy* (B) or *Five Flower Formula* (FES) can be placed on the outer part of the ear to help relieve pain and calm panicky nerves.

Essential oils are also useful in easing ear pain related to teething. Valerie Ann Worwood, author of *Aromatherapy for the Healthy Child* and *The Complete Book of Essential Oils and Aromatherapy*, suggests warming one teaspoon of olive oil and adding one drop each of lavender and chamomile essential oils (of good quality), and blending well. Soak a piece of cotton in this and use it to plug the ear.[9]

Roberta Wilson, author of *A Complete Guide to Understanding & Using Aromatherapy*, offers her recipes of either a massage (made in oil) or compress blend (made in water) with essential oils of chamomile, lavender, sandalwood and basil. The massage blend is applied on and around the ear. The compress is prepared with a washcloth and held over the ear.[10]

If the child has a stuffy nose, chances are the ear pain is a result of nasal congestion backing up into the ears. If this is the case, in addition to eardrops, a nasal spray or irrigation may be of benefit. It is important to keep the sinus passages clear so that pressure won't build up in the eardrum eventually causing pain and/or rupture. If the eardrum does rupture, be assured, that in most cases it heals quickly with no complications. *(See resources in back of book.)*

✦ *Throat* ✦

The movement of the teeth may also affect the throat. A sore, swollen or inflamed throat is quite common with the eruption of molars. It is difficult to assess whether or not a young child is experiencing a sore throat, but a loss of appetite is usually a good indication that something is wrong. A medical examination will usually confirm no real throat problems.

As the molars are coming in, children often describe a pressure or pain that radiates throughout the throat area, which is usually accompanied by either swelling, redness, headaches and/or a fever. Even if your child hasn't been affected by teething up to this point, the eyeteeth and molars may be the ones that bring some discomfort and pain. Remember certain children are sensitive to each and every tooth's eruption, whereas others aren't affected at all.

The tops of the molars are large and broad and it can take anywhere from two to eight months for them to complete the eruption process. It is not uncommon for large flaps of skin to lift up as the molar comes in, which can be very painful and annoying. Sometimes the area can get infected, creating even more pain, swelling and fever. This flap of skin may need to be professionally cleaned or trimmed off. Every situation is different.

In most cases, hygienic home care and homeopathic remedies are all you need. But your dentist and pediatrician are always a phone call away to answer questions and advise you on your individual needs.

Self-help:
If the child is old enough to gargle, a tried and true remedy for a sore throat is to gargle with warm salt water. There are also many herbal, anti-microbial and homeopathic throat sprays available that will help relieve throat pain. *(See resources in back of book.)*

The most common homeopathic remedies to relieve symptoms for ear, nose and throat problems associated with teething are:

Aconitum napellus – Sudden inflammation of the ear with severe pain; the child is fearful, restless; usually thirsty and pale; sudden sore throat after exposure to cold wind; external ear is red and hot.

Belladonna – Throbbing ear pain with a sudden onset; sudden sore throat; fever; flushed hot face; the pain is of a delirious nature and there is not much thirst.

Calcarea phosphorica – A clear, runny discharge from the nose; swollen, burning, itchy ears; diarrhea; the teeth are delayed in eruption.

Chamomilla – Ear pain in an irritable child who always complains about what he cannot have; easily angered; extremely thirsty, wants to nurse continuously; not much appetite; fever with one red cheek; gas or diarrhea.

Hepar sulphuris – An ear that is extremely sensitive to touch; ear canal is filled with white, cheesy, bloody pus; it is worse from warm applications; the mucus membranes in the nose or eyes can be involved with yellow or green discharge; sore throat with a pricking sensation that can extend into the ear; the child is irritable.

Kali bichromicum – An ear canal congested with yellow, ropelike, sticky mucus; the nose and eyes may have the same; it can take several tissues to wipe the nose clean; itchy eustachian tubes; diminished hearing; swollen glands; sinus headache; dry sore throat; postnasal drip.

Kali muriaticum – The eustachian tubes, glands or tonsils can be swollen; there is a gray or white exudation from the ear; crackling noise.

Lachesis - A constricted sore throat; usually the pain is more prominent on the left side of the throat.

Mercurius solubilis – For a sore throat with excessive amounts of saliva, drooling; pain from throat into ear; worse from heat; sweating; yellow or green nasal mucus, pus.

Phytolacca – For a sore throat when the pain is more pronounced on the right side, possibly with swollen glands.

Pulsatilla – The sad, weepy child who wants to be cared for; ear feels as if something were being forced outward, a sharp, darting pain; difficult hearing from stuffed ears; or a stuffiness of the nose with yellow discharge, a loss of smell, or a bad smell, (similar to bad breath); headache; little thirst.

◆ Headaches ◆

Most children have occasional headaches, but if they are experiencing them on a regular basis, it deserves further investigation. I suggest seeking the advice of a medical doctor to rule out the possibility of a serious health condition. Some of the more threatening reasons a child may have headaches include a tumor, meningitis, encephalitis, high blood pressure, epilepsy, or a concussion.

Once you have ruled out the threat of one of these dangerous conditions, other more basic causes can be considered, such as an exposure to toxic elements through foods or the environment, a food or environmental allergy, structural misalignment, sinus or tooth infections, fever, constipation, a hormone imbalance, low blood sugar, stress, or even teething.

Self-help:
A nutritional supplement of calcium and magnesium is wonderful for relieving a headache associated with tension. In some cases, a magnesium deficiency has even been linked to the onset of headaches. A massage oil made from a couple of drops of the combination flower essence *Rescue Remedy* (B) or *Five Flower Formula* (FES) mixed with a few drops of lavender and/or chamomile essential oils is very soothing for headaches

associated with teething. Massage over the forehead, temples and sinus area if needed. (Avoid contact with the eye area.)

The most common homeopathic remedies and flower essences for a headache associated with the teething process are:

Belladonna – For sudden onset with pounding and throbbing; the face is flushed and the head is hot, little thirst.
Bryonia – For when the pain is worse from any movement and the child's mood is like an angry bear.
Chamomilla – For irritability and whining; the child wants things then doesn't want them and is thirsty.

Combination flower essences
Five Flower Formula (FES), *Rescue Remedy* (B), *Un-stress, Tranquility* (BA), *Emergency Care* (GH)

◆ Croup, Coughs & Vomiting ◆

◆ Croup ◆

Many children will experience an attack of croup with the eruption of a new tooth. Croup is an upper respiratory infection resulting in an inflammation of the larynx, windpipe or trachea. Sometimes it involves the bronchi or air passages between the windpipe and the lungs. Its characteristic sound of a seal barking or brassiness is unmistakable and can be frightening for both the child and parent. The child has difficulty breathing and can become anxious, feeling as if he might suffocate.

(Caution: Croup is a viral infection. Its symptoms however are very similar to that of epiglottitis, a bacterial infection that progresses very rapidly and is life-threatening. The swelling can cause the air passages to be completely cut off very quickly and should be considered a medical emergency. If you are worried, call 911.)

True croup will usually last for days unless treated with a homeopathic remedy, at which point the croup sound will change into a more traditional sounding cough. The progression of the cough or cold symptoms may require additional treatment with other homeopathic remedies.

Self-help:

If the child suffers from an acute attack of croup, turn on the hot water in the shower and take her into the bathroom. Sit with the door and windows closed, creating a type of steam room. *Five Flower Formula* (FES) or *Rescue Remedy* (B) flower essence can be placed on the infant or child's physical body – anywhere. Flower essences in general can be put in water and sipped, or applied topically to the skin, as they are absorbed directly into the bloodstream. These two formulas will promote a calming or relaxing effect. The appropriate homeopathic remedy can be placed in the mouth at anytime. Stay in the bathroom until the attack subsides, the child has calmed down (usually 15 minutes) and is able to breathe. Then wrap a towel or blanket around her, cover the head and take her into a cooler room. Once the attack is under control, a cold mist humidifier placed in the bedroom will sometimes help the child breathe easier through the rest of the night. Always use common sense and dial 911 for any medical emergency.

The most common homeopathic remedies to help relieve croup associated with teething are:

Aconitum napellus – There is a sudden onset, usually in the middle of the night, after exposure to cold wind; the child is fearful.

Spongia toasta – The breathing sounds like a board is being sawed in half, and the child is anxious. This is a dry croup and the mucus membranes are usually not involved.

Hepar sulphuris – Croup with a stuffy nose and irritability; the breath may sound wheezy and is better in a warm moist atmosphere. The child is usually sweaty and may have a sour odor. This remedy is used when the first two remedies don't work.

Sambucus – Spasmatic or true croup with the attack coming on just after midnight. The child is wheezing quickly or crowing, and fears suffocation. The nose is stuffed with mucus.

Ipecac – This remedy often works when none of the other remedies have.

◆ Cough & Vomiting ◆

Coughs are very common during the teething process, especially with the eruption of the 2, 6 and 12-year molars. A cough comes in many forms – dry, shallow, persistent, occasional; with or without mucus; deep, or even congested. It all depends on the positioning of the tooth coming in and the sensitivity of the child. In some cases, the cough will come and go for months at a time and can be very annoying. Occasionally an infant or child will vomit during, or at the end of a coughing spell. Other times they might just vomit for no explainable reason. Again this type of spontaneous vomiting will most likely occur during the eruption of the 2, 6 or 12-year molars.

Self-Help:
The most common homeopathic remedies to relieve cough or vomiting symptoms associated with teething are:

Belladonna – A dry cough with a sudden onset; fever; flushed hot face; delirious nature; not much thirst.

Chamomilla – An irritable child with a scraping dry cough; whistling and mucus rattling during respiration; hoarse; continuously fussy, does not know what will make him happy; piteous moaning for what he cannot have; fever with one red cheek; easily angered; extremely thirsty, wants to nurse continuously; not much appetite; vomiting; unusual new fears.

Hepar sulphuris – The cough is either croupy or full of phlegm that can cause choking; the child is irritable; the mucus membranes in the nose are usually involved with yellow or green discharge (occasionally the eyes are affected); rattling of mucus in the chest; sensitivity to drafts; hoarseness; sore throat with a prickling sensation, which can extend into the ear.

Ipecac – A persistent dry cough; vomiting; quick, anxious breathing; cough can be so severe, the child's face may turn blue; phlegm in chest that is brought up at end of attack, usually with vomiting; better in the open air.

Kali bichromicum – A brassy or metallic sounding cough; wheezing; hoarseness; trouble expectorating a yellow rope like mucus; the nose and eyes may have the same type of discharge; sinus headache; dry, rough sore throat; postnasal drip.

Mercurius solubilis – A dry cough with excessive amounts of saliva, drooling; pain from throat into ear; worse from heat; sweating; yellowish acrid mucus in the nose or from chest.

Phosphorous – Rawness in the entire respiratory tract; the cough is dry, short, abrupt; sensation of tightness or heaviness across the chest with pain; worse at night and from cold air; sour, sweet or salty taste in mouth; sore or rough larynx; vomit; fears of death.

Pulsatilla – The child feels sad, weepy and wants to be cared for; the cough is loose during the day and dry at night; the mucus membranes of the nose, eyes or ears are involved with a yellow or greenish discharge; a loss of smell; little thirst; may be nauseous.

◆ Digestive Upset ◆

◆ Constipation, Stomachaches, Burping & Gas ◆

Digestive upset is very common while going through the teething process. Many children experience constipation, gas, bloating, burping, diarrhea or stomach pain. It is important however, to evaluate the situation responsibly to make sure the pain is not related to a serious illness. A frequent complaint during teething is pain in the stomach region, more specifically around the navel. The pain may vary in its description and intensity depending on the child. It may be a sharp, radiating, or throbbing pain. Sometimes a child may feel like he has to go potty but can't, or may feel hungry, but doesn't want to eat. In an infant, the symptoms are similar to those of colic. Usually the pain is a result of gas, but it can also be connected to a nerve pain related to the body's meridian system.

In Chinese medicine, there are meridians, or energy channels, which travel throughout the body. These meridians link the entire circuitry of the body together. Each tooth relates to a different organ in the system. Depending on which tooth is involved and whether the child is losing the tooth or a new one is erupting, he may experience different digestive upsets or pains relating to the corresponding tooth. For instance, a child losing his first tooth in the front on the bottom may endure a nerve-related tummy pain as a result of this meridian connection. *(See the chart on page 134 in chapter "Cavities & Decay.")*

Other non-medical emergency conditions that may produce these symptoms include parasites or pinworms, minor dehydration, *Candida albicans*, or emotional upset. Always use caution when determining the source of the discomfort to assure that it is not related to a more serious health condition.

◆ Diarrhea & Diaper Rash ◆

Diarrhea is another common problem during the teething process, usually accompanied by a diaper or skin rash and in some cases, a fever. Infants may experience a diaper rash, whereas an older child may get a rash elsewhere on the body. In either case the rash can be very severe with teething. In rare cases, it can even become infected.

Diaper rash associated with teething is usually due to an alkaline change in the body. This chemistry imbalance can cause the urine and feces to be more acidic, irritating the skin, and presenting a higher risk for contact sensitivity to soaps, disposable diapers and certain fabrics. Other reasons a child may experience a diaper or skin rash include a flu virus, food poisoning, exposure to a pesticide or toxic substance in the environment (i.e., a bare bottom coming in contact with a new carpet); food allergies; contact with a poisonous plant, emotional upset, or a fungus such as *Candida albicans* in the intestinal tract.

Self-help: **This section is for all digestive upsets related to teething.**
It is best to avoid dairy products when the child has diarrhea because it can aggravate the situation, even if the child is not usually allergic to them. The most important concern when a child has diarrhea, whether from teething or illness, is the threat of dehydration. It is best to give the child small sips of water or ice chips unless larger amounts are tolerated. Natural electrolyte drinks are beneficial in the prevention of dehydration and are found at most health food stores. They include Recharge, Miracle Water, etc. These electrolyte liquids replenish minerals the body has lost and will help keep the child hydrated. Dehydration can be serious and life threaten

ing if left untreated. If the infant or child is lethargic and not improving over a 24-hour period contact a qualified health care professional immediately.

Herbal teas that can help settle an upset stomach are: peppermint (not to be used in conjunction with homeopathic remedies), chamomile, slippery elm, ginger, licorice (not to be used if the child has high blood pressure) and fennel or anise. Several herbal tea companies offer a blended tea for digestive problems, such as an upset stomach, diarrhea and constipation (for the older child.)

Most doctors recommend the brat diet for diarrhea: B – banana; R – rice; A – applesauce; T – toast. You can also make a broth from cooked rice and/or barley in spring water. Use a half-cup of grain to 1 quart of water. Cook until the grain is done, and then give the child the broth.

A non-dairy lactobacillus bifidus culture (for infants to 7 years) or a non-dairy acidophilous culture (for children over 7 years) is beneficial for rebalancing the intestinal flora and can help settle an irritable bowel.

For constipation, have the child drink a lot of water. If the constipation is a result of a magnesium deficiency, NF Formulas offers a liquid calcium and magnesium (vanilla flavor) with equal ratios, for optimum benefit. Other beneficial nutrients include: Essential fatty acids, such as flaxseed oil, perilla oil, borage, etc., once or twice a day; liquid aloe vera juice (food-grade), given once or twice a day. Refer to instructions on the bottle for appropriate dosage for the child's age. *(See resources in back of book.)*

◆ *Diaper rash* ◆

If the diaper rash is the result of a fungus, pediatrician Jay Gordon, M.D. recommends a dilute solution of grapefruit seed extract and water (five drops extract to 4 ounces of water) be used as a wash for baby's bottom with each diaper change. Improvement is usually seen within a few days.

If the rash is due to an alkaline change, pediatrician Paul Fleiss, M.D.

suggests a solution of baking soda and water (one teaspoon baking soda to 8 ounces of water), also used as a bottom wash several times a day.

There are also different ointments, salves, lotions, powders, oils, etc. made from natural ingredients, which can be soothing and healing. *(See resources in back of book.)*

The most common homeopathic remedies and flower essences for digestive upset or diaper rash associated with teething are:

Argentum nitricum – Diarrhea brought on by nervous emotions or eating too much sugar, which the child craves, along with salt; stools are green, flaky, like spinach, or with mucus; excessive gas.
Belladonna – The child is restless and not relieved by a change of position; cries, delirious; green watery diarrhea; nausea, vomiting, hot red rash.
Bryonia – The child is irritable, has large, hard, dry stools and is very thirsty.
Calcarea carbonica – The child is clammy has diarrhea that smells sour; with ravenous hunger; and a moist-nettle-type rash. Or spits up or vomits after eating, loud burps, has constipation where the stool is hard at first, then pasty, then liquid.
Calcarea phosphoricum – The child with a lot of the same symptoms as *Chamomilla* with less anger and irritability; diarrhea with a lot of gas; green, slimy and hot; colicky pain in abdomen; soreness or burning around navel; vomits easily.
Carbo vegetabilis – The diarrhea is hot, profuse and involuntary; nausea, offensive gas; loud rumbling with distended abdomen and is painful.
Chamomilla – An irritable child who complains constantly; nausea, vomiting, diarrhea with green or white mucus, with colic before and during stool with temporary relief afterward; smells like rotten eggs; fever with one red cheek; easily angered.
Colocynthis – Diarrhea with violent spasmodic cutting pains in the abdomen, causing the child to bend over; better from pressure; diarrhea can be watery and yellow in color, frothy, jellylike; bilious; can be brought on after anger; irritable; intestines feel bruised; another attack comes on after food or drink.
Hypericum – Stomach pain around the navel, usually related to the loss of

the first tooth. There is usually no diarrhea involvement here. (This pain is related to the connection between the tummy and tooth meridian in Chinese medicine.)

Lycopodium – The child is bossy, has hard, small stools with ineffectual straining and a lot of gas.

Nux Vomica – The child is angry, irritable, chilled; doesn't want to be touched, has nausea, vomiting, gas, constipation or is bloated.

*Podophyllum – Diarrhea of teething children when the other common remedies have not worked, or it is of long-standing. The diarrhea is watery; can be involuntary when passing gas; a rawness or soreness of the abdomen with great weakness; made better by bending double, pressure or warmth.

Silicea – A rash that is blotchy and rose colored and the child is sweaty.

Sulphur – Diarrhea that is worse in the morning and the child must rush to the toilet upon waking; foul smell that stays with the child; loss of appetite with much thirst; aversion to being washed; rumbling colic; stools change in color; a red irritated rash; burning; cold sweat on face and feet. Sometimes this child has constipation rather than diarrhea.

* These three remedies are most commonly used for diarrhea related to teething.

Flower essences
Agrimony (B) – The child always wears a smile despite emotional problems that are then expressed outwardly though a rash.

Crab Apple (B) – The rash is due to a food or environmental sensitivity.

Combination flower essences
Five Flower Formula (FES), *Rescue Remedy* (B), *Un-stress* (BA), *Emergency Care* (GH) All of these flower combinations are for calming restlessness during stressful situations.

Healthy coat/skin (GH) – This remedy is for all types of skin issues.

Digestive Woes (GH) – This is great for all digestive concerns.

◆ Sleeplessness and Nightmares ◆

Children may experience periods of sleeplessness, constant waking, or just be inconsolable during nighttime hours while teething. Sleeplessness in children occurs for different reasons. During the infant stage the main reasons are: a wet diaper, colic/gas, hunger, fear, illness, allergies to breast milk or formula and teething. As the child gets older, nightmares, stress from the day, mineral or vitamin deficiencies, depression, anxiety, hypoglycemia, consuming foods or beverages containing caffeine, sugar, chocolate, chemicals, preservatives or food dyes can all play a role in keeping them awake at night.

Contrary to Richard Ferber, M.D., author of *Solve Your Child's Sleep Problems,* who states, "Teething pain also can cause a young child to sleep poorly for several nights, but it does not cause sleep problems that go on week after week," personal experience has proven a very different picture. I found that a child or infant's sleep patterns can be greatly influenced by the teething process, in some cases, off and on for months, especially with the eruption of molars. Again, all possibilities should be investigated to rule out a more serious health problem.

Self-help:
Aromatherapy is always a quick way of calming and relaxing a wakeful child. Some commonly used essential oils for calming are: chamomile, lavender, neroli, orange, sandalwood, thyme and ylang-ylang. Herbal teas that offer a similar effect are hops, lemon balm, chamomile, peppermint, passionflower (for children over the age of 4 years), skullcap (for children over the age of 6 years), and valerian root (for children over the age of 12 years). The mineral combination of calcium and magnesium citrate also has a calming effect on the nervous system. Give an age-appropriate dosage as recommended on bottle, before bed to help a child with a restful night's sleep. NF Formulas has a vanilla flavored liquid formula with equal ratios of calcium and magnesium. This mineral combination is also wonderful for relieving nighttime leg cramps.

The most common homeopathic remedies and flower essences for insomnia related to the teething process are:

Belladonna – The child wakes up delirious in the night possibly with pain from teething; flushed, hot head; not much thirst; may also have a sudden fever.

Calcarea carbonica – The child who is waking on a regular basis; sweating and clammy; craves eggs; night terrors; sleeps only when rocked hard.

Calcarea phosphoricum – The child is unsettled; clear discharge running from nose off and on; loose stool; gas; similar to Chamomilla symptoms with less irritability.

Chamomilla – The child wakes and wants to nurse constantly during the night; older children may have sudden fears with insomnia; nightmares; gas and irritability.

Coffea cruda – The child is in an excited, wakeful state and wants to play instead of sleep.

Gelsemium – The child feels nervous and excitable; itching on face, shoulders or head.

Passa flora – The child is wakeful and restless; in need of a quieting effect on the nervous system; hysteria.

Silicea – Insomnia with an itchy or stuffy nose; offensive perspiration; sweaty hot head; sensitive or obstinate; chilly and wants to be kept warm; constipation; night-walking; anxious dreams.

Flower essences
Aspen (B) – Heightened states of anxiety due to unknown fears.
Chamomile (FES) – The child has difficulty relaxing.
Dill (FES) – The child is nervous and overwhelmed.
Lavender (FES) – The child has overwrought nerves.
Mugwort (FES) – Excessive dreams keep the child awake.
Red Chestnut (B) – The child is constantly worrying about others.
Rock Rose (B) – Heightened states of anxiety causing nightmares.
Sweet pea (GH) – It settles nighttime tossing, turning and restlessness.
Turnera (GH) – The remedy helps regulate a child's sleep and wake time.
Vervain (B) – The child has great surges of energy.
Walnut (B) – Gives the child a sense of security and protection.

Combination flower essences
Five Flower Formula (FES) or *Rescue Remedy* (B) – Both of these flower combinations are for calming fears and encourage a relaxed state.

Chamomile (Calm Child), *Tranquility, Un-stress* (BA)

♦ Delayed Teething ♦

The timetable each infant will follow in acquiring teeth, as you already know, will vary. But if the child is 12 months old and only has one or two teeth, they would fall into this category of delayed teething.

Different reasons a child may experience delayed teething include, genetics, compromised immune function, poor nutrition, defects of the thyroid or parathyroid glands, a fibrosis (hardening) of the gums, or a vitamin D (rickets) or calcium deficiency. Children with special needs or those on prescription medications may also be delayed in teething.

A common reason for a delay in the eruption of a permanent tooth is an accumulation of scar tissue after the extraction of a primary tooth.

Self-help:
The three most common homeopathic remedies for delayed teething are:

Calcarea carbonica – The child craves eggs, vomits or spits up easily, has a sweaty head, skin (i.e., diaper rash, cradle cap, eczema, etc.), or respiratory problems.
Calcarea phosphorica – This child wants to nurse all the time, constant hunger or thirst, diarrhea, swollen tonsils, gassy, always in motion.
Silicea – The symptoms are similar to the Calcarea carbonica picture but the child doesn't like eggs; a result of scar tissue.

♦ Rhythmic Behaviors ♦

Rhythmic behaviors such as head banging or rocking can also be associated with the teething process. Other reasons a child would behave in this manner include cranial stress, frustration, a neurological imbalance or mimicking behavior.

If there is a restriction in the skull or cranium it can affect the teething process. This stops the free-flowing rhythm in which the teeth can move and grow to their full potential. When this type of restriction occurs and a child is teething, the stress that is created can prompt different sensations. Some babies grind their teeth, hit or bang their heads or repeatedly shake their heads back and forth. Others scratch, rub or pick at the ears, face, nose, etc.

When a child is displaying signs of cranial stress, a good place to start in correcting the problem is with a gentle chiropractic adjustment. Find a method that will also address the cranium (i.e., Directional Non-Force Technique, Network Spinal Analysis, etc.) or CranioSacral work (http;//www.craniosacraltherapy.org). Some children may only need one or two adjustments before their behavior and health improves. Each situation is different. If you don't see any change after a few adjustments, experiment with other modalities such as homeopathy, flower essences, nutritional supplements and counseling.

• Teeth Grinding •

Teeth grinding, or bruxism, can stem from several sources. The most common reasons are teething – especially while the molars are coming in, a nutritional deficiency (B vitamins or calcium and magnesium), a cranial restriction, low adrenal function, hypoglycemia, a hidden food allergy or parasites, such as pinworms.[11]

Hidden food allergies can trigger teeth grinding. If a child eats a food that she is sensitive to, many times it will express through restless sleep, teeth grinding or bed-wetting. Some of the more common culprits are foods containing sugar, dyes, preservatives, nitrates, chemicals, monosodium glutamate (MSG), caffeine, chocolate or artificial flavorings and sweeteners. A lot of these foods cause reactions in sensitive individuals. For example, it has been found that naturally occurring salicylates in certain fruits and vegetables can influence a child's behavior. Something as simple as grapes, cucumbers, or even apples can act as a hidden stress factor on the body.[12]

For more information on foods containing natural salicylates and their possible effects on behavior, hyperactivity, attention deficit disorder (ADD), coordination and moods, contact the Feingold Association at (703) 768-FAUS or online at http;//www.feingold.com.

Self-help:

The most common homeopathic remedies for teeth grinding related to teething are:

Belladonna – The child moans a lot and wakes from sleep with delirium; or who is always drowsy but cannot sleep; pupils dilated; eyes and face red with a hot head.

Calcarea carbonica – Teeth grinding in late teething children; offensive smell from mouth; frequent waking at night.

Cicuta – A child with the need to press the jaws together; half asleep with tossing about.

Cina – A restless sleeper; irritable and screams, needs to be in motion to be content; hacking cough; picks or rubs nose a lot.

Coffea cruda – Extreme excitability; irritability; distress; frets and worries while awake and grinds teeth while asleep.

Hyoscyamus – A child who is very talkative; laughs at everything; suspicious; dilated pupils; puts fingers in mouth continuously and presses gums together as if chewing on something.

Phytolacca – The constant desire to clench teeth; an abundance of stringy saliva; swollen glands or even throat or ear pain.

Podophyllum – The child has an intense desire to press the gums together and grinds his teeth at night. Difficult teething with diarrhea.

Stramonium – Violent grinding of the teeth; wakes in the night with fear of what is seen; outbursts of anger; continuous motion of the fingers, or hands and feet.

◆ The Mouth & Related Conditions ◆

◆ Thrush ◆

Thrush is a yeast-like fungal infection of the mouth related to *Candida albicans*. The fungus looks like a patchy white substance, similar to milk or curdled milk on the tongue, inside the cheeks and in some cases on the lips. Do not try to scrape off the substance as it may cause injury or pain to the child or infant.

If you are nursing, it is important to know that the fungus can be passed back and forth between infant and mother. It is necessary to treat both mother and child.

This condition usually occurs if a mother has had antibiotics during her pregnancy/delivery or has a systemic yeast infection herself and transfers it to the unborn baby. An infant can also get the fungus as a result of antibiotic use or poor hygiene with regard to pacifiers or bottle nipples. In rare cases it will show up after a vaccination.

Whatever the cause, having thrush can be extremely painful, and the infant is usually very fussy. He will start to nurse and then pull off because of the pain. It is important to remedy the situation quickly so the infant does not get dehydrated. The mother may get the thrush fungus on one or both of her nipples. The symptoms can include one or all of the following – tenderness, swelling, itching, redness, cracking, flaking, burning, or fever. Always contact a qualified health care practitioner for any medical questions.

Self-help:
The most common home remedies for thrush are:

• Pediatrician Paul Fleiss, M.D., suggests a mixture of a one-teaspoon of baking soda to 8 ounces of water dabbed or swabbed with a Q-tip or clean finger on the area in question, tongue, inside cheeks, etc. Always check with your physician. This changes the alkaline levels in the mouth making it a non-hospitable host for the yeast. The solution can also be used to wash the breast after each feeding to help stop the fungus from spreading.
• Pediatrician Jay Gordon, M.D., suggests a dilution of five drops of grapefruit seed extract to 4 ounces of water, swabbed on the area three or four times a day. This is very bitter tasting and some babies may protest.
•   Non-dairy *Lactobacillus acidophilous* or *bifidus* culture: The mom should take the maximum dosage, as directed on the bottle, two times a day until the bottle is gone. A nursing infant will receive a certain amount from

breast milk, but you can also supplement them by directly applying a small amount of the powder to a moistened breast before feeding. If the infant is taking a bottle, you may add the powder directly to water or formula. Make sure it is combined with a room temperature liquid and do not microwave or heat.

• A paste of the lactobacillus acidophilous or bifidous and water may also be swabbed inside of the infant's mouth on the affected area.

• Aqua Flora phase I (800-237-4100) can be mixed with a proper ratio of water and taken internally by the nursing mom, applied topically to her breast and/or swabbed in the infant's mouth with a Q-tip. (This is a liquid homeopathic for *Candida albicans*.)

• Breastfeeding moms should restrict sugar intake, limit fresh fruits and omit yeast-based breads.

The most common homeopathic remedies for thrush are:

Arsenicum album – The child is restless, yet worn out.
Borax – The child frequently lets go of the nipple while nursing, and cries from the pain; hot and tender mouth; cannot bear any downward motion.
Hepar sulphuris – The child is irritable, with white patches on the inside of the cheeks, lips and on the tongue; the base of the ulcer resembles lard.
Mercurius solubilis or *vivus* – Excessive saliva; diarrhea; swollen glands.
Salicylic acid – A child's mouth is dotted with white patches; burning, scalded feeling.
Natrum muriaticum – Thrush associated with cold sores on the lips.

• Canker Sores •

Canker sores are usually a result of stress, food allergies, poor dental hygiene or a weakened immune system. The stress of teething can definitely be a contributing factor. The sores can range in size and are found in the mouth, on the gums, inner cheeks, tongue or the inner part of the lips. Canker sores are white with a red border, and can last anywhere from two days to two weeks. They are usually very painful. Canker sores should not be confused with cold sores, which stem from a virus (see cold sores).

Self-help:

The most common herbal and nutritional supplements used to boost the immune system are:

• Hydrastis (goldenseal) mother tincture can be placed either directly on the ulcer or diluted in water and swished in the mouth. Do this two to three times a day. This particular herb does not taste very good and is sometimes better tolerated by children when a drop is placed directly on the ulcer.
• Licorice root tea also makes a soothing mouthwash and acts as an anti-bacterial and anti viral remedy.
• *A combination of goldenseal and echinacea can also be taken internally for a few days to help build the immune system. (These herbs should not be taken over long periods of time.)
• *100-200 mcg of folic acid can be added to the child's diet for the duration of the ulcer.
• *A non-dairy *Lactobacillus acidophilous* or *bifidus* culture will help rebalance the digestive tract.
• *Extra zinc, 5-10 mg, depending on the child's age, can be taken three times a week for one month to help stimulate the immune system.
• *Beta Glucan 3mg - as directed on the bottle, age appropriate.
* These are immune building supplements that can be given to the child for both canker sores and cold sores.

The most common homeopathic remedies used for canker sores are:

Borax – For sores on the inner cheeks; the mouth is hot and dry; the child cries with pain.
Calcarea carbonica – For dry mouth alternating with salivation; canker sores during teething; constipation.
Hellebore – For canker sores with an inflamed base, raised edges and that are flat and yellowish; the child's mouth gives off a fetid smell from the mouth, sometimes accompanied by swollen glands in the neck.
Lycopodium clavatum – For canker sores located under the tongue.
Natrum muriaticum – For ulcers usually found on the inner lips which cause burning pain; sensitive to hot and cold.
Nitriumc acidum – For a collection of many ulcers with a putrid smell.
Sulphuricum acidum – For a very weak child whose mouth is quite sore;

excessive amount of saliva; sores on cheeks and gums; diarrhea and sweating.

◆ *Cold Sores* ◆

Cold sores are caused by a virus in the body called herpes simplex and are contagious. The virus can be spread by touch or by sharing utensils, cups, etc. It is important for the child not to touch her eyes or genital area after touching the sore as it can cause corneal ulcers or genital herpes.

Cold sores can last anywhere from 7 to 14 days and are painful. They are usually brought on by a weakened immune system, stress, too much exposure to the sun, or from eating an abundance of foods high in L-arginine, an amino acid found in chocolate, peanuts, nuts, seeds, raw cereals, dairy, raisins, etc. These can promote growth of the virus.

Self-help:
The most common herbs and nutritional supplements for cold sores are:

• L-lysine helps fight the virus and rebalances the levels of L-arginine in the system. Give age-appropriate recommended dosage on the bottle.
• Ester C with bioflavonoids has anti-inflammatory properties and boosts the immune system; can be given two or three times a day for the duration of the sores.
• **Also see canker sores.**

The most common homeopathic remedies for cold sores are:

Carbo vegetabilis – Humid cold sores on lips and mouth; itching changes to burning when scratched; belching and flatulence.
Natrum carbonicum – Ulcers with yellow rings around them and shooting pain or burning.
Natrum muriaticum – Deep crack in the middle of the lower lip; tingling, burning and sore ulcers.
Sarsaparilla – Sores are usually found on the upper lip with a red granulated base and white borders; common during hot summer months.

✦ Herpes Simplex Virus (HSV) ✦ & Teething Difficulty

In 1992, a study at the University of Texas Health Science Center in San Antonio, examined two groups of teething infants – Group A: 20 infants experiencing teething difficulty and Group B: 20 infants in no apparent distress. The groups were tested for the presence of herpes simplex virus (HSV) to see if there was any correlation between the virus and teething difficulty. Nine infants in Group A were positive for HSV. Infants in Group B were all negative for HSV and showed no other symptoms of teething difficulty.[13]

In a generation where the herpes simplex virus is so prominent, this study offers a small amount of food for thought as to why teething discomfort appears to be more of a problem for children today.

✦ Coxsackie Virus ✦

The coxsackie virus, also known as hand-foot-and-mouth disease, is an upper respiratory infection marked by small red or white blister like bumps in the mouth, on the tongue, feet, hands and fingers. In rare cases, I have even seen the blisters spread to other parts of the body such as the arms, legs and head.

It is primarily a childhood disease, but has been known to infect some adults. The first clue a child may have the virus comes from a complaint every time he eats or drinks. Blisters usually start in the mouth and are extremely painful. They last anywhere from seven to 14 days and are often accompanied by a fever. The virus is contagious and can be transmitted through bodily excretions – saliva, coughing, sneezing, feces and contact with the sores themselves.[14]

Hand-washing and separate towels are a must. Do not share food, drink or utensils. The child should be kept away from other children until all the blisters and symptoms are gone.[15]

Two possible complications a child may encounter are dehydration, because most children refuse to eat or drink when they have the blisters in their mouths; and the blisters on the tongue spread back towards the throat making swallowing and breathing difficult. Always consult a physician for medical emergencies.

There is no specific treatment in Western medicine for coxsackie but there are a few homeopathic remedies that successfully shorten the duration of the virus and ease the pain.

Traditionally the virus lasts up to two weeks (in rare cases, longer). But if the appropriate homeopathic remedy is given, in most cases the virus will be gone within 24-48 hours, or at least be well on its way.

Years ago, if a child had the coxsackie virus once, they would become immune. But in recent years, the virus' pattern has become recurrent. Children are now getting it three or more times.

Self-help:
The most common homeopathic remedies and flower essences used for the coxsackie virus are:

Capsicum – The blisters spread and have a stinging pain when touched by food or drink; bad smell from mouth; thirsty.
Natrum muriaticum – The mouth feels dry but is not; blisters sting and burn when touched by food.
Phosphorous – Blisters that are extremely painful; the child craves cold drinks or ice chips, but cannot tolerate them due to the pain; excess saliva; pale and exhausted.

Combination flower essences
Five Flower Formula (FES) or *Rescue Remedy* (B) – Both of these flower combinations are for calming fears and encourage a relaxed state.
Chamomile (Calm Child), *Tranquility, Un-stress* (BA)

• Behavioral & Emotional Reactions •

A child's mood, behavior and emotional state can be strongly influenced by the process of teething. Heightened states of anxiety, e.g., social anxiety, fear of separation, being alone, the dark, an elevator ride, etc., low self-esteem, or out-of-control verbal or physical behavior, can all be byproducts of a tooth's eruption.

The volatility of these emotions or actions can be dramatic. One minute the child may be balanced, sweet and focused, the next minute she is crying, screaming and throwing things. A simple question or event can send the child into an irrational state, where coherent communication is virtually impossible. Some children display restlessness or sadness, are fidgety or angry, throw things, bite, hit, kick, swear, scream, display a Dr. Jeckle and Mr. Hyde personality, trouble concentrating and/or show signs of depression. Others have described their feelings physically and emotionally as wanting to jump out of their skin or just have an overall uneasy feeling inside. Fortunately all of these emotions and behaviors respond well to homeopathic and flower essence treatments.

Self-help:
The most common homeopathic remedies and flower essences for behavioral and emotional reactions to teething are:

Aconitum napellus – For heightened states of fear, panic, performance anxiety, etc.
Belladonna – When there is caged, animal like behavior, red cheeks, biting, dilated pupils with moaning.
Calcarea carbonica – The child has a lot of anxiety, digestive problems, depression, and is sweaty or clammy to the touch.
Calcarea phosphorica – Try this remedy if the child is having similar symptoms to the Chamomilla picture, but had no response with the remedy.
Chamomilla – The child is irrational, whining, impatient, fearful, fidgety, restless, gassy, biting and is having nightmares.
Cina – This remedy is again similar to Chamomilla, but with more screaming, extreme rudeness and overall nasty behavior.

Iodum – The child has to be busy all the time or he becomes anxious, with sudden impulses to violence.

Lycopodium – For a loss of self-confidence, afraid to be alone and fear of new social situations, yet bossy towards parents.

Natrum muriaticum – For depression with fatigue and anger.

Phytolacca – For a teething child with the irresistible desire to bite the teeth together.

Flower essences

Aspen (B) – The child is experiencing unknown fears.

Elm (B) – The child feels inadequate and overwhelmed in general or by their responsibilities.

Chamomile (FES) – This child has changeable moods and fluctuating emotions that are usually accompanied by stomach problems.

Cherry Plum (B) – The child feels out of control of his emotions or body.

Chicory (B) – The child wants to control everything or everyone, and be the center of attention.

Crab Apple (B) – There is self-judgment and low self-esteem.

Feverfew (GH) – The child is experiencing deep emotional feelings or depression with anxiety or restlessness.

Gentian (B) – The child has a negative outlook and is depressed.

Gorse (B) – The child feels completely hopeless and is mistrustful.

Impatiens (B) – The child is very impatient.

Joe Pye Weed (GH) – The child feels like he is drowning in responsibility.

Larch (B) – The child lacks self-confidence and fears failure.

Marrow (GH) – This child is scared to grow up, common at any age, but especially during adolescence.

Orange (GH) – Constant rage or stormy temper tantrums are a sure sign for this remedy.

Vine (B) – If the child is inflexible, aggressive and contrary.

Willow (B) – The child has resentment, anger and a negative mental attitude.

Combination flower essences

Five Flower Formula (FES) or *Rescue Remedy* (B) – Either of these remedies will help a child who feels out of control of his body or emotions, has panicky fear, is impatient, irrational, is sad from grief or having trouble concentrating.

(BA) *Un-stress, Calm Child, Transform Anger, Tranquility.*

(GH) *Anxiety, Emergency Care, Outburst.*

✦ Attention Deficit Hyperactivity Disorder ✦

The two most overlooked reasons why a child might be experiencing symptoms described as attention deficit hyperactivity disorder (ADHD) or attention deficit disorder (ADD) are leaky gut syndrome and the influence of the teething process.

Leaky gut syndrome occurs when the wall of the small intestine is damaged and toxins (yeast and large molecules), such as incompletely digested fats, proteins and starches, seep through the walls into the blood-stream. An overgrowth of yeast and parasites commonly accompanies leaky gut syndrome. The syndrome can trigger food allergies (when the immune system attacks the undigested food particles), environmental allergies and malabsorption of important nutrients, all of which have an influence on behavior and result from (and contribute to) a weakened immune system.

According to *Insight Magazine*, ADHD and ADD have been categorized as a mental illness "which is diagnosed when a child meets six of the 18 criteria described in the *Diagnostic & Statistical Manual of Mental Disorders* or *DSM-IV*, published by the American Psychiatric Association, or APA."[16]

Where did this mental illness originate, and why is our society dealing with such a large epidemic among our children today? In 1987, the APA deter-mined by a vote that these symptoms would constitute a state of "mental" illness called ADHD.[17] Some of the symptoms include not paying attention in school, trouble concentrating, distractibility, impulsiveness, aggressive behavior, not listening when spoken to directly, failing to follow directions, losing things, forgetfulness, fidgeting with hands and feet, talking excessively, blurting out answers, difficulty awaiting a turn, even poor motor coordination.[18]

Interestingly, many of these symptoms describe a child experiencing a food or environmental sensitivity, or a teething child. Perhaps this diagnosis is simply a misinterpretation of what is really going on with a child? In the United States alone, there are nearly 6 million children between the ages of 6 and 18 that have been diagnosed. One report by the United Nations revealed that 3 to 5 percent of all schoolchildren in the United States are taking the prescription drug Ritalin.[19] Ritalin is classified as a schedule II narcotic by the Drug Enforcement Administration, which puts the drug in the same category as opium, morphine and cocaine – the most addictive in medical usage.[20]

Some of the known side effects of Ritalin are loss of appetite, insomnia, tics or Tourette's syndrome, headaches, stomachaches, increased heart rate or blood pressure, social withdrawal, irritability, moodiness, short-term growth retardation, suicide, depression, irrational acts of violence and murder.[21]

Many children take Ritalin Monday through Friday and go off the drug on the weekend. Unfortunately, this abrupt cessation of a schedule II narcotic has prompted what is referred to as "Sunday suicides." There were quite a few reports of children hanging themselves, most of which took place on a Sunday after being off the drug for two days.[22] Even the American Psychiatric Association states in its *Diagnostic and Statistical Manual* that the major "complication" of withdrawal from Ritalin is suicide.[23]

Another alarming statistic is that in the past 10 years, most of the shooting sprees and senseless acts of violence in our schools have a common denominator – the child responsible for the action was taking a prescription psychiatric drug, including the 1998 shooting spree at Springfield High School in Oregon by 14-year-old Kip Kinkel. He was reportedly taking Prozac and Ritalin. Another familiar case is the 1997 rape and murder of a 7-year-old girl in a Las Vegas restroom by 18-year-old Jeremy Strohmeyer. He had also been diagnosed with ADD and was prescribed dexedrine.[24]

Self-help:

One of the most effective ways to correct leaky gut syndrome in children over 5 years, is through a group of products by Renew Life – Kids Paragone, Kids Parazyme and Fiber Smart. To get more information on these products go to http;//www.renewlife.com.

The most common homeopathic remedies and flower essences for the symptoms of ADHD or ADD related to the teething process are:

Arsenicum album – Restlessness (at times they want to crawl out of their skin) and fearfulness.

Calcarea carbonica – Anxiety, delayed teething, sweaty and clammy, may crave eggs, trouble sleeping.

Calcarea phosphoricum – Symptoms similar to the Chamomilla picture, but that remedy hasn't worked.

Chamomilla – The child is irritable; has a sensitive nervous system, headache, diarrhea, tired, gassy, complains all the time.

Cina – Child is cross, irritable, screams, has nightmares, picks at his nose, scratches his bottom; prone to teeth grinding. Parasites can also be a causative factor.

Lycopodium clavatum – Child likes to be in control (a reversal in the parent-child command), spacey, fear of being alone and new social situations, digestive problems, craves sweets, hypoglycemic tendencies, lacks self-confidence, constipation, can't sit still, and all symptoms are worse between 4:00 - 8:00 p.m.

Natrum muriaticum – The shy, introverted child craves salt; can be inappropriately disruptive but feels terrible about his behavior and fears making mistakes.

Plantago major – A child is hasty or hurried in her work, desires to do several things at once, but does not complete them; restless, nervous and confused.

Tarentula hispanica – Rhythmic behavior, tapping, drumming, dancing; mischievous, hurried, impatient, destructive, impulsive and distractible.

Veratrum album – The child is precocious, restless, may display repetitive behaviors, is debative, bossy and always busy; exhibits inappropriate touching, kissing or hugging.

Flower essences

Bottle Gentian (GH) – The child has difficulty with concentrating and focus.

Clematis(B) – Lives in a daydream state.

Cosmos (FES) – The child is overwhelmed by too much information at one time.

Elm (B) – The child is overwhelmed by his responsibilities and therefore can't concentrate.

Feverfew (GH) – The child is hyperactive, restless, and shows signs of being depressed.

Filaree (FES) – The child is obsessed with (sometimes unimportant) details.

French Marigold (GH) – The child has trouble processing what is being said.

Indain Pink (FES) – The child is easily influenced by other activities around them.

Lemon (GH) – The child needs more energy and clearer thinking to have a better understanding of what is being taught.

Madia (FES) – The child has trouble focusing on details, and is easily distracted.

Pumpkin (GH) – The child is a procrastinator and has trouble getting things done.

Rabbitbrush (FES) – The child is inundated by too many details and activities at once.

Scleranthus (B) – Indecision prevents him from learning.

Vervain (B) – The child has too much physical or mental energy to sit still.

Walnut (B) – The child needs protection from outside surroundings.

White Chestnut (B) – Persistent unwanted thoughts cloud his mind.

Combination flower essences

Rescue Remedy (B) or *Five Flower Formula* (FES) – Calms and centers a child.

Inspiration (BA) – Promotes a balanced state for better problem solving.

Mental focus (BA) – Stimulates improvement of attention, concentration and learning ability.

Perfect balance (BA) – Helps restore mental & physical coordination.

Un-stress (BA) – Establishes clear, focused and positive thinking during stressful time.

Anxiety (GH) – The child is too anxious to settle and learn.

Conclusion

Any of the symptoms discussed in this chapter could be the result of an infection, virus, food poisoning, flu, a neurological problem, appendicitis, parasites, etc. The situation should be investigated thoroughly to be sure the symptom is not an indication of a more serious health problem and that the child receives all the proper medical attention necessary. Once it has been established that it is indeed a simple illness, possibly related to teething, then you can explore the benefits of a more natural healing process. When in doubt, always seek the advice of a trained medical professional.

"*I think the tooth fairy is made up – maybe they are one inch tall. How are they going to carry all those coins? Maybe they have a car or they won't be able to deliver the money. The Tooth fairy is someone who takes our teeth and puts money instead. They do their job at night when everybody is sleeping. They do it because they collect our teeth. She has our key to open the door and looks under our pillow.*"

Edgardo – 8 years old

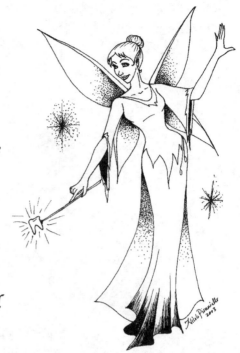

"*I think the tooth fairy looks beautiful because she has a pink dress. She looks like a movie star and has soft skin, but dry and is cold. Well, she takes our tooth and puts a dollar. She puts them at night when we are sleeping. Also she turns small and takes the tooth. She does it in our bedroom. Then she makes a necklace with the teeth and wears it to parties.*"

Anna – 6 years old

"*First the tooth fairy looks like a little flying woman with wings on her back and has a magic wand. Second, the tooth fairy feels like a normal person. Third, she acts nice because she gives us money. I like the tooth fairy. She is friendly and makes us happy. Children make her happy too. First, she gets to your house with her wings. Second, she goes to your house when your tooth is under your pillow. Third, she lives at a tooth castle. Finally, I'm happy when she comes.*"

Jessica – 8 years old

Chapter Five

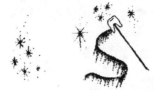

Cavities & Decay

◆ Tooth decay. How it happens! ◆

Dental cavities and caries are multi-causal and cannot be attributed to any single factor. We know that if you don't brush your teeth and see the dentist for regular cleanings, you will get cavities. But tooth decay is not that simple. Following the recommended dental care still leaves many children with cavities. There are several different internal and external factors that play a significant role in the development of tooth decay.

Different lighting systems can even have an impact on dental caries in children. A two-year study conducted in Canada in the late 1980s proved this point when a group of schoolchildren was exposed to different lighting systems. Students receiving light from full-spectrum fluorescents with ultraviolet light supplements developed less decay over time than those who were not exposed to the UV rays. Thus, ultraviolet light served to reduce the development of cavities. The students that received the ultraviolet light supplement also demonstrated better attendance, the greatest gains in height and weight and the best academic achievement. Warren Hathaway, a psychologist and one of the authors of the study, speculates that ultraviolet light stimulates the production of vitamin D in the skin, which in turn affects calcium metabolism and contributes to better dental health.[1]

Other external causes include the positioning of the teeth in relation to each other, exercise, hygiene (bacteria/food/medicines in the mouth), brushing technique and stress. Internal causes include heredity, diet, tooth hardness, hormones, physical illness, prescription medications, vitamin and mineral absorption and the direction in which fluid is transported through the teeth. All these factors play a part in creating dental cavities.

◆ When You Are Pregnant ◆

Few people realize that dental health begins at conception. As the fetus begins to develop in the first trimester of pregnancy, teeth also begin to grow. The mother's mineral and vitamin balance is extremely important during this time, as it contributes to the formation and mineralization of her baby's teeth. If there is a deficiency during this first phase of development, the results cannot be reversed.

◆ Morning Sickness/Illness ◆

If the mother experiences severe morning sickness or becomes ill during pregnancy (i.e., severe nausea, vomiting, dehydration or fever), the strength of a child's tooth and its susceptibility to decay can be influenced. For instance, a fever during pregnancy can cause an imperfect mineralization in the baby's teeth. Stephen Moss, author of *Your Child's Teeth: A Parent's Guide to Making and Keeping Them Perfect*, describes the process, "If the woman gets a fever from a virus or some other infection (a common occurrence between the fifth and ninth month of pregnancy), the delicate balance of calcium and phosphorus salts in her bloodstream could become upset. This would affect the quality and quantity of tooth structure that is forming in the fetus. The disruption will continue for as long as it takes for the mother's system to regain its balance." The results of the illness on the child's dental health can only be assessed after the teeth erupt. Moss also states, "An infectious illness or a high fever affects the adjustment of calcium and phosphorus salts in the baby's bloodstream. The teeth mineralize imperfectly. Poor enamel and dentin crystals form, causing the teeth to be more susceptible to decay."[2]

There is also a higher rate of decay in premature babies. If the expectant mother gives birth before term, it is possible that the child's teeth will be affected. There is evidence that full-term children have fewer cavities. The reason for this is simple. Certain areas of the teeth mineralize around the time of birth. If a baby is born prematurely, these areas may be more susceptible to decay.[3]

Another condition that may arise in premature babies, or in a child with a systemic defect such as cerebral palsy, is enamel hypoplasia. The characteristics of enamel hypoplasia are similar to bottlemouth syndrome. The difference is that this condition is evident as soon as the tooth emerges. With bottlemouth syndrome, the teeth erode over time.[4]

Morning sickness is a common occurrence during the first few months of pregnancy. F. Batmanghelidj, M.D., author of *Your Body's Many Cries for Water – You Are Not Sick, Just Thirsty*, describes morning sickness as a sign of dehydration. He states, "During the intrauterine stage of cell expansion, water for cell growth of the child has to be provided by the mother." So if the fetal tissue is not receiving what it needs, it will express this deficiency through the mother's body, thus creating morning sickness. Another contributing factor to morning sickness is related to an increase in hormonal activity, which produces a chemical byproduct that builds up in the body. Proper hydration and daily walks can be helpful.[5]

Self-help:
There are safe and effective herbal and vitamin formulas to assist during this stage of pregnancy, as well as products designed to stimulate appropriate acupressure points to relieve nausea. *(See resources in back of book.)*

The most common homeopathic remedies for nausea or vomiting during pregnancy are:

Arsenicum album – Vomiting with exhaustion, thirsty, but drinks only in sips, and usually feels chilly.
Carbo vegetabilis – The woman gags while she talks, has low energy and craves cold carbonated drinks.
Cocculus – Symptoms that worsen from riding in a car, or smelling or thinking of food, with a tendency toward insomnia from emotional excitement or from headaches.
Ipecacuanha – Nausea or vomiting with a lot of mucus or saliva.

Nux vomica – A sour taste with nausea; worse in morning and after eating; or she has to vomit but cannot; irritable and may be constipated.

Phosphorus – Nausea or vomiting that is relieved when given cold water or ice chips; but once the fluid becomes warm in the stomach it is vomited up; craves ice cream; extremely weak and fearful.

Pulsatilla – Nausea with intolerance of warm rooms; better outside or with windows open, emotionally sensitive, little thirst, cannot tolerate rich or fatty foods.

Sepia – Nausea that is intensified by the smell or thought of food which is usually preferred, symptoms can be temporarily relieved by eating; there is an ambivalence about friends, loved ones, even the pregnancy itself. The woman is usually irritable, selfish and occasionally dizzy.

Veratrum album – Violent vomiting alternating with diarrhea; there is much thirst and hunger; and the person is weak and chilly.

Combination flower essences
Five Flower Formula (FES), *Rescue Remedy* (B), *Un-stress* (BA), *Emergency Care* (GH) All of these flower combinations are excellent for calming stressful situations.

Always consult a medical practitioner before taking any medications during pregnancy.

♦ Bottlemouth Syndrome ♦

Bottlemouth syndrome is the uncontrollable decay of upper primary teeth that occurs in infants as a result of drinking formula or juice from a bottle. Drinking a bottle at bedtime allows the liquid to pool in the mouth and sit on the teeth for many hours. A bottle enhances the dripping of liquid into the baby's mouth, even when there's no sucking, surrounding the upper teeth in a bath of enriched carbohydrates. If you are using a bottle to give naptime or nighttime comfort to your child, it is important to be aware of the consequence of decay.

The physiology of breastfeeding and its milk composition are quite different than bottle and formula. Consequently, breastfeeding contributes to this condition only in rare cases, when the frequency of night nursing is almost continuous.

There is only a small amount of supporting evidence substantiating a link between breastfeeding and dental caries. The breast is much more pliable and is therefore pulled into the back of the mouth. The milk is let down and ejected in response to the baby's sucking action and swallowed through a reflex that is triggered automatically. The infant must continue to suck the breast for the milk to keep flowing. Once the baby stops sucking, so does the flow of milk. Therefore, the milk is not allowed to pool in the infant's mouth. To insure that no milk is leftover in the mouth, when he is finished nursing gently move him with a rocking motion. La Leche League International (LLLI) states, "A small percentage of at-risk breast-fed children develop dental caries in spite of breastfeeding, not because of it."[6]

Premature babies are also susceptible to enamel hypoplasia, which is a condition similar to bottlemouth syndrome. This condition is common in premature infants and in children with systemic defects such as cerebral palsy.[7]

♦ *Diet: Sugar Equals Cavities* ♦

All decay-causing bacteria thrive on sugar. By eliminating sugar from the diet, the tooth-decaying germs have less chance to breed.

There are three important factors when looking at the correlation between sugar and tooth decay – what types of food are eaten; the frequency of consumption; and how often you brush. For example, if you drink soda (even the natural kind) all day long, you produce plaque activity most of the day. This can put the health of your teeth in jeopardy. A smarter choice would be to have the drink close to a meal, then brush as soon as possible. Let's say you enjoy eating jellybeans or licorice. These foods stick to the teeth and sit there for long periods of time. If you eat these sticky foods as an afternoon snack and then brush your teeth, but continue to drink soda throughout the day, the soda will be the bigger offender.[8]

Back in the 1930s, Weston Price, D.D.S., honored dental research specialist and author of *Nutrition and Physical Degeneration*, spent decades studying the nutritional aspects of teeth and their structure. He visited an isolated island twice during a 15-year period. During his first visit he was delighted to find the natives had no tooth decay. However, on his second visit, he found half the teeth of the islanders had rotted away. After further investigation, Price found that sugar and white flour had been brought to the island in trade for one of the island's treasures. Eventually, the traders lost interest and did not return. That is when the islanders reverted back to their native diets, saving what was left of their teeth. Price states,"It was as if an epidemic of decay had hit the people, then went away, allowing the half-decayed teeth to heal."

In the mid-to-late 1950s, Ralph Steinman, D.D.S., of Loma Linda Dental College in California began to present his research and concepts, which would further substantiate Price's theory about the correlation between diet, sugar and tooth decay. Many experts think that acid levels are partly responsible for creating a decay prone environment. Steinman found that on a healthy diet, more acid was produced than in a high-sugar diet. Yet the teeth observed on the sugar diet showed etching on the enamel surface, whereas in a healthy diet there was no visible etching. Steinman concluded that decay was more of a systemic problem coming from within the body. Obviously, other factors also play a role, but they are not the initiating factor. Steinman and Price shared the same theory: the hardness of enamel is not related to a tooth's resistance to decay.[9] (This opinion is not shared by all practitioners in the field of dentistry.)

Steinman confirmed this theory in studies conducted with rats. He found that the decay appeared whether the rats ate the food by mouth or were fed through the stomach. When Steinman injected a substance (i.e., sugar) into the abdominal cavity, within minutes it traveled up to the solid structure of the rats' teeth. This study provided tremendous insight into understanding the process of decay in relation to the mechanics of the body.

◆ *Butter vs. Margarine* ◆

Price also observed that there was an increase of mineral absorption when butter is part of the diet. His research showed that there was a resistance to decay associated with an unknown fat substance (with similar characteristics of the fat-soluble vitamins A and D) present in butter. Confirming Price's findings, Hal Huggins, D.D.S., noted that children had healthier facial form and tooth positioning when they were raised on butter rather than margarine.

◆ Gum Chewing ◆

Gum chewing can also be a contributing factor in the development of dental caries. Television commercials have been promoting gum chewing to freshen breath for years, and more recently, for cleaning teeth when brushing isn't convenient. However, George Meinig, D.D.S., author of *"New" Trition – How to Achieve Optimum Health* and *Root Canal Cover-Up*, says that gum chewing has its drawbacks and is an influential factor in the development of temporomandibular joint (TMJ) disorder, excessive wear to tooth enamel and an imbalance of the digestive enzymes that are produced by the pancreatic gland, disrupting proper digestion.[10]

As for the commercials, chewing gum is only a temporary measure in the prevention of bad breath. It is important to take a look at what the underlying causes of bad breath really are and to correct them – eating odorous food (i.e., garlic, onions, etc.), a systemic infection (i.e., sinus or intestinal) or poor hygiene (i.e., not brushing regularly or gum disease).

In terms of teeth cleaning, gum chewing can be of some benefit if used in moderation when brushing isn't convenient. The increased flow of saliva that is created, along with the agitation of the gum substance against the teeth, helps remove some food particles. So, if you are going to encourage your child to use this method occasionally, suggest using a brand that is sugarless. Meinig also states, "Bathing the teeth repeatedly with sugar, whether from gum, candy or food, provides bacteria nourishment. And the acid byproducts of bacteria cause hard tooth enamel to dissolve."

There are two types of gum – regular and sugarless. Regular gum contains approximately half a teaspoon of sugar in every stick. Not only does sugar contribute to tooth decay but it also affects bones and other tissues, leading to osteoporosis, arthritis and other degenerative diseases.[11] Sugarless gums may be better for you compared to regular gum, but they too have risks.

For instance, they contain chemical sweeteners – sorbitol, manitol, xylitol, phenylalanine, saccharin and/or hydrogenated glucose syrup (still a sugar), plus artificial flavors and colors, that over time can be toxic and polluting to the body. Gum made with saccharin actually has a warning on the package stating that saccharin has caused cancer in laboratory animals. *(See chapter on "Hazards, Cautions & Emergency Situations.")*

◆ Hygiene ◆

Dental hygiene, along with diet, functions as one of the best preventive measures a parent can teach a child. Good hygiene practices should start at birth. The best way to start is by using a simple gentle massage technique with a clean finger or a moist gauze pad several times a day, which helps gum circulation and the environment of the mouth by minimizing oral bacteria and the overall acidity levels.[12]

Experiment with different routines and positions as the baby grows to find what works best for your individual needs. With infants, the process can be an extension of nursing or bottle-feeding and may be incorporated into the feeding ritual.

As children get older, it can become more of a game. Some families combine oral hygiene with bathing, by brushing while in the bathtub. Pediatric dentist, Kevin Hale states, "Teeth should be brushed as soon as they erupt." Remember that you are building the foundation for the future of your child's teeth.

If you keep a close eye on a child's teeth from the time of eruption you should be able to detect a decay problem early. This is an important part of your job as a parent. The enamel on an infant's tooth is not as thick or hard as a mature tooth. Decay can move very quickly, so regular examinations are important. During the first few years these exams can be done at home unless you suspect a problem. Once all the baby teeth are in, a trip to the dentist's office is in order.

◆ Environmental & Food Allergies ◆

Both food and environmental allergies play a role in tooth decay. Food allergies increase the mouth's acidity and vulnerability to tooth decay. Food and/or environmental allergies can produce chronic nasal congestion and mouth breathing. If the child is continuously breathing through the mouth, the saliva production will be reduced, leaving the mouth dry. This condition deprives the oral cavity of the naturally protective enzymes produced in the saliva.[13]

◆ Medications ◆
Over-The-Counter, Prescription & Homeopathic

The oral consumption of medications can be another contributing factor of tooth decay. Prescription medications, either liquid or chewable (i.e., antibiotics, asthma, seizure, cardiac, etc.), over-the-counter medicines (i.e., nighttime cold, decongestants, etc.), and homeopathic remedies are quite often given at bedtime after the teeth have been brushed. Most of these medications include some sort of sweetening element. Sucrose is the primary sweetener, and levels ranging from 25 to 60 percent have been found in these products.[14] Even a large percentage of homeopathic remedies are administered on a sugar pellet, all of which need to be cleaned off the teeth.

Cough drops or throat lozenges bathe the teeth as long as they are held in the mouth and continue to exert influence until the teeth are brushed. Chewable vitamins and medications can get lodged between teeth. Liquid vitamins and medications coat the teeth. It is best to give medications and vitamins around mealtime and then follow with a good brushing. If it is necessary to administer them between meals or at bedtime, encourage brushing as soon as possible. Many homeopathic practitioners prefer you use a mint-free toothpaste while under their care because mint can cancel out the remedy in sensitive individuals.

Another problem is encountered with children who are on certain prescription medications for attention deficit hyperactivity disorder (ADHD), seizures, lupus, diabetes, etc. Some of the medications prescribed for these conditions will deplete the body of minerals, and/or interfere with their absorption influencing a tooth's strength and susceptibility to decay.

♦ Exercise and Stress ♦

Exercise is instrumental in the generation of bone growth and strength, so it is essential for a child to participate in a regular exercise program. Stress also influences the overall health of the child, including teeth and gums. Help support your child's well-being by giving him tools to assist in coping with the many stresses of his day.

Self-help:
There are herbal combinations or calming teas for kids of all ages that will help reduce stress levels. *(See resources in back of book.)*

Flower essence

Elm (B) – If the child is completely overwhelmed by his responsibilities this essence can be combined with any of the other combination flower essence.
(Also see flower essences in chapter "Natural Remedies for Teething-Related Symptoms," section on Behavioral & Emotional Reactions.)

Combination flower essences
Five Flower Formula (FES), *Rescue Remedy* (B), *Un-stress* (BA), *Emergency Care* (GH) Any of these flower combinations are excellent for calming stressful emotions.

♦ Bacterial Plaque ♦

Bacterial plaque is a thin film, which covers our teeth and is a combination of bacteria, food and saliva with different pH levels of acidity. When saliva and bacterial plaque are combined with certain foods, a weak acid called lactic acid, is formed. Even though saliva helps neutralize this acid, when lactic acid gets under the bacterial plaque and encounters a tooth, decay forms. This acid substance eats through the enamel of the tooth, then into the dentin and, if left untreated, down to the pulp.

There are beneficial and harmful bacteria in every person's mouth. The bacteria-containing deposits found on a tooth are comprised of a large population of microorganisms that stick to the hard enamel surfaces of the teeth. There are more of these one-celled organisms in your mouth than in any other place in your body.

The largest percentage of bacteria found in plaque is composed of *Streptococcus* (this variety does not cause strep throat). Several theories exist about the effect of this variety on dental health. One theory is called the Specific Plaque Hypothesis (SPH), which maintains that *Streptococcus mutans* (one of the bacteria) plays a key role in enamel caries. *Streptococcus mutans* attach to the hard surfaces of a tooth for colonization. These bacteria produce an extracellular enzyme, which forms plaque and hastens sucrose fermentation. When the total cell count of *Streptococcus mutans* is high, it offers an alluring environment for dental caries.

The primary ingredient that allows *Streptococcus mutans* to sustain and multiply is sugar. These harmful bacteria thrive on sugar. In 1960, Keyes and Fitzgerald demonstrated that dental decay was a transmissible infection due to *Streptococcus mutans*, and the extent of the infection was found to be sucrose-dependent. The development of smooth-surface caries on molars or incisors is most often seen in individuals who consume sucrose frequently or who have a low salivary flow.[15]

◆ *The Correlation Between "Fluid Flow,"* ◆ *Hormones & Cavities*

The movement of fluid or "fluid flow" through a solid tooth is very important in the prevention of tooth decay. The fluid flow moves from the pulp chamber through the dentin, then the enamel and into the mouth. This is considered an outward fluid-flow, which protects teeth. If there is a disruption in the endocrine system and hormone level, it causes an inward fluid flow or reversal of this protecting action by sucking bacteria, acids and other damaging agents in the mouth, back into the tooth.

This inward fluid flow happens in response to an imbalance of the parotid hormone, which is controlled by the hypothalamus, a master gland located in the brain. Certain foods have the ability to stop the hypothalamus from functioning properly by altering hormone levels. This in turn creates an inward, fluid flow precipitating tooth decay. These foods include refined sugar and fast foods.[16]

◆ Crowded Teeth ◆

Children with overlapping, crowded or crooked teeth need to be extra cautious about keeping their mouths clean. Teeth that are positioned incorrectly create little pockets that collect food and bacteria. Therefore, it is important to take extra measures to clean the teeth properly. Spend a little more time brushing, flossing, water irrigating and/or flushing. This added effort will greatly improve chances for healthy teeth and gums throughout life.

◆ Heredity ◆

In part, the health of a child's teeth is also determined at conception by genetic heritage. This map of the past involves genes passed down through generations to you and your spouse, then by both of you to your child. These genes influence the quality of blood supply, growth rate, hormone output and the jaw and tooth size, all of which affect the possibilities of your child's rate of tooth decay and gum disease.

In some cases there are rare genetic diseases involved, causing mouth abnormalities. Harelip or cleft lip and cleft palate fall into this category. Cleft lip is a failure of developing parts of the embryonic lip to meet and grow together. Seventy percent of those who have a cleft lip also have a cleft palate. A cleft palate is when there is no separation or divider between the roof of the mouth and the nose. This can be hereditary, but 80 percent of the time, it is the result of drug use, including the steroid hormone cortisone and meclizine (a motion sickness drug), certain vitamin deficiencies or X-rays. The developing fetus is most vulnerable in the first few weeks or months of pregnancy.

✦ *Genetic Errors* ✦

If there is an error in the gene development, several problems can occur. They include: a congenital overgrowth of gum tissue (hereditary ginguial fibromatosis), mottling or other disorders of the tooth's hard outer shell or enamel (hypophosphatasia, amelogenesis imperfecta, dentinal dysphasia), congenital absence of some or all teeth, various bone disorders affecting the jaw and/or jaw joint as well as the bite.

Some other genetic diseases, syndromes or inherited medical conditions which could affect the mouth are diabetes, hemophilia, hereditary vitamin D-resistant rickets, Fanconi's syndrome, pseudohypopara-thyroidism, Hurler's syndrome, Rh incompatibility, congenital porphyria and Hutchinson's disease.[17]

Hutchinson's disease is caused by an injury to the tooth-forming organ during development. It affects the central incisors with a narrow crown at the edge and a notching in the center. It is sometimes seen in patients with a history of congenital syphilis.

Opalescent dentin is a hereditary trait carried by a gene and affects the quality and quantity of dentin produced by the forming cells. These teeth wear down excessively with chewing stress. Normal translucency is replaced with a dull opal color.

Extra care should be given and emphasized in children with special needs. Children with CCD (congenital cardiac disease) are more susceptible to endocarditis from oral infections. Enamel hypoplasia is common in CCD children.

Other genetic patterns include: a permanent tooth that doesn't develop, two rows of teeth or supernumerary teeth, a permanent tooth locked in the bone (ankylosis), or hereditary oral tori (a growth of bone in the jaw or palate or benign tumor.)

♦ When To See A Dentist ♦

The three best weapons against tooth decay are good hygiene – brushing your teeth to reduce bacterial plaque; eating a good diet – eating fewer foods that form acids rapidly, like sugar and fast foods; and routine cleanings – scheduling routine cleanings and check-ups for your child. This will give teeth the optimal attention they need for a lifetime.

Parisa Ezzati, D.D.S., says it is important to have good oral hygiene habits from birth, but suggests, "Most children don't need to see a dentist until around the age of 3 years, when they have all their primary teeth – unless of course there is a concern before then." Other situations may warrant earlier dental visits, such as dental abnormalities, or the case of a child who is medically compromised, on certain prescription drugs, taking oral medications regularly, or is developmentally delayed.

An introduction to the dentist should take place before there is a problem, so the child will not associate the visit with struggle or pain. The first appointment should be about establishing a relationship between child, dentist and parent, exploring the office and equipment, sitting in the chair, seeing what some of the tools and gadgets do, and counting teeth. Most dentists will gift the child with a toothbrush and/or a small toy, making the experience enjoyable.

Ezzati also recommends a return visit once a year for a cleaning and exam, which is usually all that is needed, provided there are no special circumstances. The yearly visit allows a dentist to keep a close eye on developing teeth and the opportunity for early identification of a problem. Choose a dentist that you trust, one who responds well to questions. Your questions can be the discerning factor in saving your child from unnecessary work, vs. appropriate measures. Early detection, nutrition and hygiene are the best prevention against future decay.

What To Do if Your Child Has Dental Cavities: Decay and Treatment Options

If decay does occur in a primary tooth, it needs to be treated immediately to prevent pain and infection. In severe cases the infection can even affect the jawbone. The primary teeth act as a guide for the permanent teeth so it is important to keep baby teeth healthy. If a primary tooth has to be pulled due to decay or infection, it is important to preserve the space to prevent nearby teeth from wandering out of position. This can cause a problem for the permanent tooth when it is ready to come in, because it may not have enough room.[18]

The treatment of a cavity depends on the severity of decay. Usually, a cavity requires the removal of the decay and the application of a filling substance to the cleaned area. This seals the site, reconstructs the tooth and protects from further decay. If it is a minor or shallow cavity, the process of repair can be easy. The dentist can use an air abrasion machine, which blows pressurized air and tin oxide into the area, thus avoiding the use of a drill. There will be cases however, that will require drilling. This is where creative thinking comes into play. Many children can be talked through a procedure, or are easily distracted by listening to headphones with their favorite music. Depending on the child or situation, the preparation process may necessitate some type of local anesthetic or oral sedation to proceed with the work. Some of the different options include numbing the gum topically, anesthesia through injection, nitrous oxide (laughing gas) or oral sedation.

According to Ezzati, kids are usually responsive to conversation. If Ezzati runs into a problem, she might use a small amount of nitrous oxide or laughing gas mixed with oxygen to help calm the child. The mixture does not linger. The sedation stops immediately. Ezzati states, "I have found that a lot of times children become anxious under the influence of local anesthesia." Certain local anesthetics contain epinephrine, which can cause an accelerated heart rate, anxiety and/or sweating.

If your child requires a local or general anesthetic, it is important to know the risks and cautions involved. After a local anesthetic, do not let the child eat until the effects have worn off. There is a danger of biting the tongue, cheeks, or lips without feeling pain. *(See chapter on "Hazards, Cautions & Emergency Situations.")*

Tooth decay eventually leads to root canal infections and other health problems. If the decay involves the nerve of a primary tooth, a child will need a pulpotomy, which involves the removal of the upper portion of the nerve. A pulpotomy is performed on newly erupted teeth where the roots have not completely formed, either in a primary or permanent tooth. This procedure allows the roots to continue developing undisturbed. Sometimes a stainless steel crown is used to finish the job. If the infection is in a permanent tooth however, and the root system is fully formed, a root canal may be necessary, in which case it is important to fully understand the risks involved.

A focal infection is created when germs from one part of the body move to another part. "Ninety-nine percent of the focally infected diseases arise from the tonsils or teeth," says Dr. Frank Billings, Dean of the Faculty and Professor and Head of the Department of Medicine, University of Chicago. Bacteria become trapped in teeth and tonsils, and produce diseases elsewhere in the body.[19]

Meinig, one of the 19 dentists who organized the Endodontic Association, wrote *Root Canal Cover-Up*, about Weston Price's 25-year research program on this subject. Price worked with 60 of the nation's leading scientists, and the program was conducted under the protection and support of the American Dental Association and its Research Institute. He looked at how the bacteria in teeth metastasize (similarly to cancer cells) to other parts of the body, infecting other organs, glands, or body tissues.

His findings confirm teeth that have undergone root canal work and have been filled always remained infected. The infection resides in the tubes or tubules inside the dentin. There are so many tubules in each tooth that if you placed them side by side, they would extend for three miles.[20]

When an infection needs root canal treatment and the filling is placed, the bacteria are sealed in the tubules. Price proved that medications used to sterilize the root canal had no effect against the bacteria found in dentin tubules.

The bacteria found in dentin tubules are anaerobic, which means they do not need oxygen to survive. They are also polymorphic – they mutate or change form and thrive in the absence of oxygen. When sealed in, they seek a new route out and seep through the cementum and alveolar process, eventually selecting an organ, gland or tissue as a new home. Most dentists think antibiotics are able to control all focal infections, which come from teeth. Meinig states, "To date, none of the more than 100 drugs used in treating root canals has been capable of penetrating the miles of dentin tubules."[21]

When this metastasis happens, other physical manifestations take place, creating disease in other parts of the body. Price demonstrated this conclusion repeatedly through human and animal observations and studies. Chronic constitutional conditions cleared up immediately when the tooth of infection was pulled. His findings encompassed a wide range of illnesses such as imbalanced blood pressure, heart, respiratory or urinary conditions, colitis, arthritis and much more.[22]

In Chinese medicine, there is a connection between teeth and different organs. If you take this into consideration, Price's observations make sense. For instance, on the lower teeth, the kidney and bladder correspond to the central and lateral incisors. This urogen system also affects ears and sinuses, which corresponds to the symptoms most infants experience when they are getting their first teeth. The 6-and 12-year molars on the bottom relate to the lung, large intestine, bronchial tubes and sinus. Physical symptoms in these areas (i.e., coughs, diarrhea, sinus) are the ones that most commonly occur as these molars erupt. *(See chart on next page.)*

◆ *Fillings* ◆

There are four substances that can be used in filling a cavity – amalgam, composite resins, gold and porcelain. When my generation visited the dentist, our cavities were routinely filled with amalgam, but today there are other choices.

134

The Connection Between Teeth, Body Organs & Tissue Systems

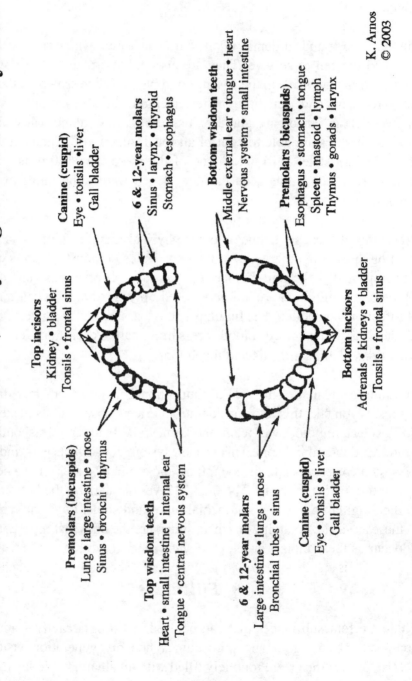

Top incisors
Kidney • bladder
Tonsils • frontal sinus

Canine (cuspid)
Eye • tonsils •liver
Gall bladder

6 & 12-year molars
Sinus • larynx • thyroid
Stomach • esophagus

Bottom wisdom teeth
Middle external ear • tongue • heart
Nervous system • small intestine

Premolars (bicuspids)
Esophagus • stomach • tongue
Spleen • mastoid • lymph
Thymus • gonads • larynx

Bottom incisors
Adrenals • kidneys • bladder
Tonsils • frontal sinus

Premolars (bicuspids)
Lung • large intestine • nose
Sinus • bronchi • thymus

Top wisdom teeth
Heart • small intestine • internal ear
Tongue • central nervous system

6 & 12-year molars
Large intestine • lungs • nose
Bronchial tubes • sinus

Canine (cuspid)
Eye • tonsils • liver
Gall bladder

K. Arnos
© 2003

Amalgam

Also known as silver or mercury fillings, amalgam is a mixture of metals including silver, mercury, copper, tin, zinc, and occasionally nickel. Even though it is stronger than composite and porcelain, according to current research, amalgam comes with a high toxic price tag. Organic mercury compounds are among the most potent developmental nerotoxicants, which can cross over the placenta, cause kidney damage and more. Herbert L. Needleman, M.D., states, "We are conducting a vast toxicologic experiment in our society in which our children and our children's children are the experimental subjects."[23]

The mercury in amalgam fillings continuously releases toxic vapors in the mouth at low-level concentrations when subjected to the pressure and a brasion of chewing. To give you a better idea of the toxic levels amalgam fillings produce, Richard Casdorph, M.D. and Morton Walker, D.P.M., the authors of *Toxic Metal Syndrome* state, "Vapor escaping from dental amalgam fillings offers more mercury poisoning than eating contaminated fish, being exposed to latex wall paint, and drinking polluted water."[24] Obviously, this is not preferable as a filling substance. *(See chapter on "Hazards, Cautions & Emergency Situations.")*

Composite Resin

Composite resin is a material made from a combination of plastic resin and filler made of finely ground, glasslike particles. When the mixture hardens in the cavity, its color is similar to the color of the tooth itself. This is the material of choice for filling a child's cavity.

Porcelain

Porcelain fillings are made of a ceramic material and are also called porcelain inlays. This material is not very practical for use in a child's mouth because it is made to order at a laboratory. The use of porcelain filling requires two visits to the dentist and the cost is similar to that of a gold inlay.

Gold Inlays

Gold inlays are also made at a laboratory. They last the longest, have the highest durability factor and are the most expensive of the four choices.

But again, gold is not practical for filling a child's tooth.

✦ *Dental Sealants* ✦

Dental sealants are synthetic coatings made up of different plastic chemicals. The thin plastic coating is applied primarily, but not exclusively on the chewing surfaces of the back teeth. The focus is on the back teeth/molars because they have irregular surfaces with pits and grooves, which tend to trap food and bacterial debris.

Most dentists recommend applying dental sealants as soon as the permanent teeth erupt. The theory is that this thin plastic coating will meld into the pits and grooves of the teeth, sealing them so that bacteria cannot multiply and cause decay.

To apply dental sealants, the tooth being sealed is cleaned and then dabbed with a very mild acidic solution, whose properties are similar to that of vinegar or lemon juice. This process slightly roughens the tooth's surface so the sealant will bond to it properly. However, sometimes the sealants don't bond properly and come off. They can also wear off in certain areas. In either case, they need to be checked periodically to ensure efficiency. If necessary, they can be reapplied.

At first glance one might think of dental sealants as a miracle. But in the past few years, a study conducted by researchers at the University of Granada in Spain uncovered a controversial side to this wonder coating.

So before you routinely have a dental sealant applied to your child's teeth to help prevent cavities, be sure to read the chapter on *"Hazards, Cautions & Emergency Situations."* It is our job as parents to do as much research as possible before going with the flow. Even if the advice comes from an authoritative person, that person may not have all the facts.

◆ Teeth Staining Or Discoloration ◆

The most common reasons an infant or child's teeth are stained are from too much fluoride, prescription drugs and food. If an excess of more than 2ppm (2 parts fluoride per million parts water) of fluoride is ingested during certain stages of the pregnancy, the developing fetus can develop a condition known as "mottled teeth." Evidence of this overuse can present itself as an opaque white discoloration or a brownish stain of the enamel. In severe cases, pitting with brown or chalky stains appear and sometimes become crumbly in consistency. *(See chapter on "Fluoride.")*

If certain antibiotics are taken during pregnancy, they are passed through the mother's bloodstream to the unborn child's blood. The antibiotic is then deposited into the developing teeth (and other areas). The evidence usually shows up as a discoloration of the tooth – yellow, gray or brownish. The main culprits are tetracycline, doxycycline and minocycline, all members of the tetracycline class or group. This staining of the teeth can also occur in a child after birth as a result of taking these antibiotics. The stain itself is not dangerous.

Teeth may also become stained from food. This staining comes from the naturally occurring color of the food itself. Fruit berries are one of the worst culprits for staining teeth, especially blue-, black- and boysenberries. Beets are another vibrant-colored vegetable that causes discoloration. Fortunately, the staining of teeth through foods can usually be remedied with a good brushing as soon as possible.

Teeth also have blood vessels, which are located in the pulp chamber and extend through the roots via canals. If there is a trauma to a tooth, one of the blood vessels may rupture (hematoma) causing a brown, gray or black color to appear through the translucent enamel. And last but not least, if a woman contracts German measles (rubella) during pregnancy, there may be imperfect enamel formation, expressed through a discoloration of a tooth or teeth.

Conclusion

There are many contributing factors in the development of dental cavities, which is why good habits such as a healthy diet, personal oral hygiene and exercise are essential in developing strong healthy teeth.

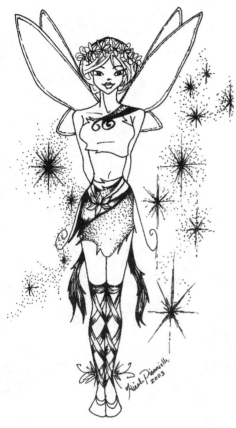

"I lost a tooth when I was eating corn on the cob. My dentist gave me a little box called the tooth treasure box and I put my teeth in the box.

Once upon a time there was a little fairy, not just an ordinary fairy, the tooth fairy. She collected teeth because they were like little corn chips to her. She eats them. A tooth under the pillow is like a super-market where she can buy the chips. That is why she leaves you money. The tooth fairy is dressed in a beautiful dress that has all kinds of colors. She has an antenna on top of her head and wings to fly around at night. She is almost like nocturnal because once and a while he has to fly in the daytime. She lives far, far a way. She knows when the kids have lost their teeth because she has this little TV with channels. When she clicks on the channel it shows, who has lost their teeth, on what day and the location of the house."

Anna – 8 years old

"My tooth felt very wiggly and I kept fiddling with it until it fell out. Then I put it under my pillow and the tooth fairy took it and put it in her castle. It is in Washington, D.C. and is called the White House. They call it the White House because they put teeth in it and they are white. It is a huge, huge, big tooth and lots of fairies live in it. There is a store next door where there is a lot of money – that's where the fairies get the money to put under the pillow."

Ben – 8 years old

Chapter Six

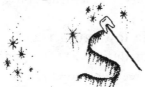

Fluoride: Friend or Foe

Most people know fluoride as the cavity fighter of our time and are unaware of the controversy surrounding its use. The possibility that fluoride might be dangerous or even poisonous to children seems utterly preposterous to most people, but when I started researching the subject, I was shocked. *The Clinical Toxicology of Commercial Products* calls fluoride, "more poisonous than lead and just slightly less poisonous than arsenic."[1]

Children ingest fluoride in many forms: They drink fluoridated water and other drinks made from this water, e.g., sodas, juices, etc.; and they eat foods that have been grown with or prepared with fluoridated water; they use products that contain fluoride, such as toothpaste, mouthwashes, multivitamins, fluoride tablets, treatments and rinses.

Prior to its use in water, fluoride was respected for its toxic properties. In high concentrations, it was a standard ingredient in rat and roach killer. Some physical symptoms from fluoride poisoning include stomach and gastrointestinal tract problems, loss of appetite and fatigue. In certain instances, it has caused death.[2]

The ideal amount of exposure recommended by the American Dental Association (ADA) for optimal health is 1ppm (part per million) or one milligram of fluoride in one liter of water. This recommendation was established back in the 1940's. According to the ADA, the American Academy of Pediatrics Interim Policy and the American Academy of Pediatric Dentistry (AAPD), the fluoride supplement schedule as of 1994 showed the dietary supplement dosage for children as: birth-6 months = none, 6 months-3 years = 0.25ppm, 3-6 years = 0.5ppm, 6-16 years = 1ppm and after 16 years of age, dietary supplementation is no longer recommended.

These figures are specific to the understanding that there are no other means of fluoride ingestion during the same time period. The ADA states, "Ingestion of higher than recommended levels of fluoride by children has been associated with an increase in mild dental fluorosis (spotting or discoloration) in developing, unerupted teeth."[3]

The original dosage of 1ppm was based on the assumption that the average person consumes between one and two quarts of water per day. It is recommended that people drink eight glasses of water a day, which is the equivalent of two quarts. But today most people drink more than that, especially those who live in warmer climates, pregnant woman and children. Children drink more water in relation to their body weight than adults, which gives them a greater chance of exposure and susceptibility to toxic pollutants. Generally they are also more active and require additional hydration. During pregnancy, the recommendations are even higher. But since many water systems have fluoride added, as do other beverages, children are most likely receiving more than the established safe amounts.

◆ A Brief History Of Fluoride ◆

Who made fluoride the cavity fighter of our time? In 1939, C.J. Cox, a biochemist working at the Mellon Institute in Pittsburgh, voiced his enthusiasm for the use of fluoride in water to help prevent tooth decay. The Mellon Institute, which also owned the Aluminum Company of America (ALCOA), had assigned Cox the task of finding a use for the waste product sodium fluoride produced by the aluminum and phosphate fertilizer plants. In addition, there were 50 other industries that also wanted to get rid of their toxic waste. Unfortunately, conclusive studies had not yet been completed, and claims regarding fluoride were spoken without studies substantiating its effectiveness in the prevention of cavities.

Another strong voice was that of Oscar Ewing, an attorney who worked for ALCOA. Ewing eventually became one of the head figures at the U.S.

Public Health Service. This put him in position in 1950 to formally endorse the fluoridation program. Then Edward L. Bernays jumped on the bandwagon. Dubbed by the *Washington Post* as the "father of public relations," Bernays' biggest triumph was the promotion and success of the government fluoridation campaign.[4]

Fluoride is the only chemical added to U. S. municipal water used to mass medicate, rather than to render water safe to drink. It is not an essential nutrient. And it has never received approval from the U. S. Food and Drug Administration (FDA). Rather, it is listed as an "unapproved new drug," and the Environmental Protection Agency (EPA) lists it as a "contaminant".[5]

In 1993, it was John V. Kelly, a New Jersey State Assemblyman that discovered that fluoride had never been approved by the FDA, as required by law since 1938.[6] Kelly's investigation revealed that neither the FDA, nor the AAPD, nor the National Insurance of Dental Research had proof of fluoride's safety and effectiveness. Kelly states, "Parents are spending millions of dollars annually on products that have not been proven effective. They then have to spend millions more to repair the fluorosis caused by these products."[7]

◆ *Dental Fluorosis/Mottling* ◆

One of the first visual signs of fluoride poisoning is mottling of the teeth, also known as dental fluorosis. In mild cases of mottling, chalky white areas are seen on the tooth. In more advanced stages there are yellow, brown or black stains. The teeth can also develop pits, crevices and tips that are prone to break off easily.[8]

John Yiamouyiannis, author of *Fluoride: The Aging Factor*, contends that dental fluorosis is a permanent record that shows fluoride has interfered with the basic life functions of the enamel-forming cells (ameloblasts), causing them to produce damaged collagen.

Collagen is the most abundant of all the proteins in the body, making up 30 percent of the body's protein. If there is a disturbance to collagen, the skin, ligaments, tendons, muscles, cartilage, bones and/or teeth can all be in jeopardy. Data suggest that fluoride can lead to an irregular formation of collagen in the body.[9]

Fluoride also invades tissues and organs, damaging biologically important chemicals called enzymes. This disturbance can also lead to a wide range of chronic problems such as: muscular and skeletal weakness, premature aging of the bones, rheumatoid or osteoarthritis and cancer.

In areas where drinking water is fluoridated, the health of the people is affected. One of the first cities to be fluoridated in the U.S. was Newburgh, New York. In 1945, John Caffey, a professor of clinical pediatrics at the College of Physicians and Surgeons, Columbia University, co-authored a report about X-ray examinations being made of the children in this area. Caffey noted cortical defects in the bone X-rays of 13.5 percent of these children, as compared to 7.5 percent in a neighboring town, Kingston.[10]

In Bartlett, Texas, research done in 1943 and 1953 indicated that using fluoride in the drinking water at a ratio of 8ppm increased the mortality rate to more than three times higher than that of a neighboring town, which used a lower amount of fluoride. Interestingly, the U.S. Centers for Disease Control and Prevention and the Safe Water Foundation indicate that 30,000 to 50,000 excess deaths are observed in the United States each year in areas that add fluoride to the drinking water at a ratio of 1ppm.[11]

Another problem with fluoridated water is that toxicity levels vary in hard and soft waters. According to James Benfield, D.D.S., fluoridated soft water proved to be more toxic than fluoridated hard water. Referencing a case "in one area of India where the fluoride level was about 3ppm, and the water was soft, there was greater toxicity with respect to dental and skeletal fluorosis than in another area where the concentration was 5 to 6ppm of fluoride, but the water was hard." Yiamouyiannis states, "The softer the water, the more fluoride passes through the intestinal wall."

Benfield also explains that fluoride is a compound and when boiled, becomes more concentrated or toxic. If you are using fluoridated water for cooking be aware that the concentration levels rise and present more of a danger in the water and in the foods being cooked.

Other studies on 9-year-old children from China, Argentina, Great Britain, Italy and Japan showed an incidence of severe dental fluorosis as fluoride levels increased above 1ppm. This was also the case with similar studies done in the United States with a slightly older age group (11-13 year olds). Environmental, growth and nutritional information also has to be taken into consideration in the evaluations. Yiamouyiannis' book gives impressive representation substantiating dental fluorosis in children 9 years and older in charts showing cities and states; numbers of children; the amount of fluoride in drinking water (ppm); and the percentage with dental fluorosis or mottling teeth. These charts were compiled from investigations led by H. Trendley Dean of the U. S. Public Health Service and published in 1937.[12]

Consider these chronological highlights on recommended fluoride dosages in Yiamouyiannis' book:

> • *"In 1977 the Fluoride Symposium of the 143rd annual meeting of the American Association for the Advancement of Science and again in 1978, the Journal of the American Dental Association reported that 0.5 mg fluoride supplements were causing dental fluorosis. But nothing was done about it and millions of children have been poisoned as a result.*

> • *In the 1978 Physicians' Desk Reference (1,637), the following statement with regard to fluoride supplements was made: "A daily fluoride intake of 0.5 mg from birth to age three-years...is recommended."*

> • *In the 1983 Physicians' Desk Reference (1,977), the following statement with regard to fluoride supplements was made, "In communities with less than 0.3 ppm fluoride in the water supply, the recommended dosage is 0.25mg daily between birth and two years of age." (Editor's note: the recommended dose had been cut in half in just five years.)*

• In the 1992 Canadian Dental Association Proposed Fluoride Guidelines, the following statement was made: "Fluoride supplements should not be recommended for children less than three-years-old."

• In 1993, thanks to the tenacity of a New Jersey legislative aide, Michael Perrone, the FDA was forced to admit: 1) that they have no studies showing that fluoride tablets or drops are either safe or effective in reducing tooth decay and 2) that the sale of fluoride tablets and drops is illegal."

◆ Fluoride & Fertility ◆

The FDA examined countries that had 3ppm of fluoride in the water. It found that women aged 14 to 49 years had decreased total fertility rates associated with increased fluoride levels.

This was documented by Stan C. Freni, a scientist at the FDA, in an article that originally appeared in the *Journal of Toxicology and Environmental Health*. Freni also adds that as of 1994, animal studies have shown that fluoride affects fertility in most animal species.[13]

◆ Fluoride During Pregnancy ◆

In a report published in the *Journal of Dental Medicine*, Vol. 16, October 1961, "Prenatal and Postnatal Ingestion of Fluorides – 14 Years of Investigation – Final Report", Dr. Reuben Feltman of Passaic General Hospital in New Jersey, observed that 1 percent of his patients (pregnant women and children) could not tolerate the recommended supplementation of 1mg of fluoride per day and experienced symptoms such as headaches, gastrointestinal disturbance, skin disorders, eczema, itching and dryness of the throat.[14]

An examination of cattle on Cornwall Island gives a better understanding of the more serious toxic effects of fluoride and pregnancy. In published findings by Dr. Lennart Krook, Dean of Post Graduate Research at Cornell

University, *Cornell Veterinarian Newsletter*, April 1979, he reports:

"Chronic fluoride poisoning in Cornwall Island cattle was manifested clinically by stunted growth and dental fluorosis to a degree of severe interference with drinking and mastication. Cows died or were slaughtered after the third pregnancy. The deterioration of cows did not allow further pregnancies."[15]

In the book *Tooth Fitness*, Thomas McGuire refers to a hypothetical pregnant woman who drinks two quarts of fluoridated water a day, plus other beverages made from fluoridated water, i.e. juice, tea, etc. The woman also eats foods high in fluoride, such as seafood, especially shellfish, ready to eat cereals (i.e., corn flakes, grapenuts, etc.), brushes her teeth with fluoride toothpaste, and rinses with fluoride mouthwash. McGuire suggests the woman would be ingesting approximately 5mg or more of fluoride a day, which is more than any arguably safe maximum dosage.

Consequently, if a child were consuming this much fluoride, he too would be ingesting excessive amounts of fluoride. This could put a child who is in the enamel-forming stage of tooth development into a high-risk category for mottling. McGuire suggests that this over fluoridation process may be responsible for an increase of mottling in the past few years.[16]

In studies published in the *Journal of the American Dental Association* (Dec. 1995, July 1996, July 1997) on pervasive overexposure to fluoride due to "the widespread use of fluoridated water, fluoride dentifrice, dietary fluoride supplements and other forms of fluoride...(there is) an increased prevalence of dental fluorosis, ranging from about 15 to 65 percent in fluoridated areas and 5 to 40 percent in non-fluoridated areas in North America."[17]

After reading the information in Yiamouyiannis' book (Chapter 8, "Genetic Damage") I believe the use of fluoride during pregnancy to be an extremely high-risk behavior, and think all parents owe it to themselves and their children to do their own research and formulate their own decisions.[18]

✦ Intelligence Quotient (IQ) ✦
& The Central Nervous System

Recently Joel Griffiths and Chris Bryson authors of "Fluoride, Teeth and the A-Bomb," *Earth Island Journal*, Winter 1997-98, obtained World War II documents that included declassified papers about the Manhattan Project, the U.S. military group that built the atomic bomb.

The authors state, "The papers reveal that fluoride was a key chemical in atomic bomb production. Millions of tons of fluoride were needed to manufacture bomb-grade uranium and plutonium for nuclear weapons throughout the Cold War. One of the most toxic chemicals known, fluoride rapidly emerged as the leading chemical health hazard of the U.S. atomic bomb program – both for workers and nearby communities."

The papers also mention a Manhattan Project memo dated April 29, 1944, which states, "Clinical evidence suggests that uranium hexafluoride may have a marked Central Nervous System (CNS) effect ... It seems most likely that the F [fluoride] component rather than the T [code for uranium] is the causative factor."

As far back as World War II, there was enough evidence to support the approval of an animal research project to study the effects of fluoride on the CNS. Unfortunately, the information seemed to disappear and no evidence of the Manhattan Project's fluoride/CNS research could be found in the files.[19]

In the early 1990s, Phyllis Mullenix and other researchers from Harvard Medical School, Eastman Dental Center, Iowa State University and Forsyth Research Institute conducted the "first laboratory study to demonstrate that CNS functional output is vulnerable to fluoride, that the effects on behavior depend on the age at exposure and that fluoride accumulates in brain tissue."[20]

The 1995 paper published in *Neurotoxicology and Teratology* brought to light the unsettling possibility of a link between fluoride and its effects on the central nervous system.

Mullenix writes, "Experience with other developmental neurotoxicants prompt expectations that changes in behavioral function will be comparable across species, especially humans and rats. Of course behaviors per se do not extrapolate, but a generic behavioral pattern disruption as found in this rat study, which can be indicative of a potential for motor dysfunction, IQ deficits and/or learning disabilities in humans."[21]

In China, human research was done to study the effects of fluoride on children's IQ and CNS. Chinese investigators found that high levels of fluoride in drinking water (3-11ppm) affect the CNS directly without first causing the physical deformations of skeletal fluorosis.

In 1995, the *International Journal of Fluoride* reported a study that measured the intelligence of 907 children 8 to 13 years of age, where the fluoride levels in the environment fluctuated. In areas where there were higher levels of fluorosis, I.Q. levels were lower than in areas that had less fluorosis. The study authors noted that the development of intelligence appeared to be adversely affected by the different amounts of fluorosis the children were exposed to within their environment.[22]

Roger D. Masters, a professor emeritus of government at Dartmouth College, found that people who drink water treated with silicofluoride tend to absorb more lead. In one of Masters' studies, he found that residents of 25 Massachusetts communities who used silicofluoride were more likely to have elevated levels of lead in their blood than were residents of 25 other Massachusetts communities that did not.[23]

Masters' findings also concluded that lead poisoning affects the child's developing brain, and even at low levels, cuts the child's IQ and causes learning and behavior problems.

• Delayed Teething •

In Frank Murray's book, *The Big Family Guide to All the Minerals*, he quotes Albert Schatz, a professor of emeritus at Temple University, "Teeth erupt later in fluoridated children than they do in non-fluoridated children of the same age. That delayed eruption, which is well documented, has several interesting implications. Children who have fewer teeth in their months obviously have fewer teeth that can decay." Schatz also points out that when teeth erupt later, there is a lower decayed-missing-filled (DMF) ratio, even if fluoride does not prevent cavities.[24]

◆ Acute Cautions & Hazards ◆

You may have never thought of your tube of toothpaste as a hazard to your child's health. But in Yiamouyiannis' book, he quotes Procter and Gamble, in regard to a 7-ounce tube of fluoride toothpaste, as saying, "Theoretically at least, it contains enough fluoride to kill a small child."[25]

Most children will not ingest a whole tube of toothpaste. But it can be pretty tasty, thus very inviting to a child. So even if children only sample it, it still can be hazardous to their health. According to research, one-hundredth of an ounce of fluoride can kill a 10-pound child, and one-tenth of an ounce can kill a 100-pound adult. Twenty percent of children, 1 to 2 years of age, ingest 0.25mg of fluoride simply by brushing their teeth. Four-to 6-year-olds consume 25 to 33 percent of the toothpaste on their brush.[26]

In 1997, poison control centers in the United States received over 12,000 calls regarding fluoride poisoning and children. Toothpaste and mouthwash ingestion were the main sources.[27] Symptoms of fluoride poisoning can be more or less serious depending on how much is ingested. Some examples are nausea, vomiting, diarrhea, abdominal pain and fatigue (as a result of the inhibitory effect on thyroid activity). In rare cases, children have died.

When Danielle was 3 years old, I took her to a pediatric dentist. After cleaning her teeth the dentist gave her a fluoride treatment. I never considered that this simple dentist-recommended procedure could be dangerous. A year later I read Yiamouyiannis' book. He cites one case in the *New York Times* from January 20, 1979 regarding the death of William Kennerly, a 3-year-old boy. After a routine teeth cleaning, the child received a fluoride treatment from the dental hygienist, who mistakenly did not give proper instruction on the rinsing procedure. Instead of rinsing the fluoride out of his mouth with the water, the child drank it and died hours later.

Yiamouyiannis also points out that there have been other accidental fatal overdoses. Surveys have shown that in over 6 percent of children receiving treatments, nausea and vomiting were reported either immediately or within hours after the treatment.[28]

If you do keep a bottle of prescription fluoride tablets in the house, make sure it is locked up and out of reach, as it can be fatal. Infant/children's liquid multivitamins with fluoride should also be stored safely. Some kids love the taste of these, and if given a chance might consume the whole bottle.

◆ Sudden Infant Death Syndrome (SIDS) ◆

Sudden infant death syndrome or SIDS, is the sudden unexpected and unexplained death of an infant. The cause to date is uncertain, but research suggests different contributing factors may play a role in the syndrome. For instance, in February 1992, Glen S.R. Walker reported in the *New Zealand Medical Journal* that a connection had been made in Australia between SIDS and cities that had the highest rate of fluoridated water.[29]

◆ Fluoride In Our Foods ◆

The mineral fluorine or calcium fluoride naturally occurs in many foods. Sodium fluoride (waste produced by the aluminum, uranium and phosphate fertilizer industries) is the substance that is supplemented in our drinking water, etc. There are many foods that are naturally low in fluoride: fresh vegetables, fruits, nuts, meat, whole-grain cereals and dairy products, depending on where the products are grown and whether the irrigating water, or water given to the animals is fluoridated.

Foods containing high amounts of fluoride include seafood, especially shell fish, salmon, mackerel, sardines, and popular breakfast cereals, such as Corn Flakes and Grape Nuts.[30, 31]

The smartest way to avoid high levels of fluoride in your food is to eat at home as often as possible and as purely and simply as possible. If you live in an area that has fluoridated water, you may be eating soups, drinking tea, coffee or consuming other delectables made with fluoridated water. In February 1997, the Academy of General Dentistry (AGD), representing 35,000 dentists, warned parents to limit their children's intake of juices due to excessive fluoride content.[32]

◆ *Who Is Fluoridating Water?* ◆

According to *The Big Family Guide to All the Minerals*, the following countries have never used fluoridated water, or have discontinued its use for legal or other reasons: Austria, Belgium, Denmark, Egypt, France, Germany, Greece, Holland, India, Italy, Luxembourg, Norway, Spain, and Sweden.

Conclusion

Children are being exposed to excess amounts of fluoride in many ways: Pediatricians are prescribing multivitamins with added fluoride; dentists are prescribing fluoride tablets; some restaurants, depending on what city you live in, are cooking with fluoridated water; certain sodas and juices are made with fluoridated water; most toothpaste is supplemented with fluoride and more, so by the end of a day no one can accurately calculate how much fluoride a child has ingested. The role of fluoride needs to be seriously re-evaluated in relation to the health and well-being of our children.

"My mom pulled my tooth with a Hello Kitty cloth – it just popped right out! I was really surprised. So I put it under my pillow and asked the tooth fairy for a dog and some money. But then I fell asleep and never saw her. I know she has a little pink dress, a wand, wings to fly and oh yes, a pen – she wrote me a note about my second tooth. She told me she was sorry she couldn't give me the cat I wanted. She takes the teeth to Tooth Fairy Land where she has a collection in a tunnel. She watches you, so she knows when the tooth falls out, and then she comes. The tooth fairy is very small and it takes four fairies to move the pillow. Tooth Fairy Land is way up in the sky."

Ireland – 6 years old

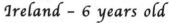

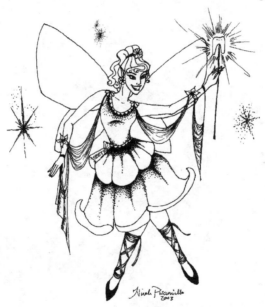

"My first tooth fell out when I was getting ready for school, eating a waffle. I took a bite and there was something hard in the waffle. I spit it out and it was a cracked tooth. The tooth fairy lives up in the sky and wears a white sparkling gown that doesn't show her feet. She has sparkles all around her long, blond hair. I wonder why she doesn't come in the daytime. And I know she doesn't come through the front door because the alarm doesn't go off. She gives the teeth to the new babies so they will have them."

Melissa – 8 years old

Chapter Seven

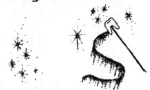

Hazards, Cautions & Emergency Situations

Technological advances made over the past 15 years are amazing, but we've also created a hazardous environment in which we are exposed to hundreds of unnoticed, almost invisible pollutants daily. These toxins can have a cumulative effect on our health and the health of our children.

Many of these poisons are found in unsuspecting places including cleaning solutions, both household (oven, floor, carpet, clothing, window, air, etc.) and personal care (mouthwashes, toothpaste, deodorant, creams, etc.); substances or procedures used in dental or doctors' offices (fillings, sealants, X-rays, fluoride, etc.); gardening products (pesticides, insecticides, herbicides, fertilizers, etc.); and even foods (preservatives, chemicals, food dyes, etc.). The list of everyday contaminants is long, and can negatively affect children and their teeth.

◆ Oral Teething Solutions ◆

Teething solutions are for external use on the gums of a teething infant. You apply a small amount on the tip of your finger or Q-tip and rub it into the gum tissue. It has an analgesic affect that relieves pain when a tooth is getting ready to erupt. Most of the solutions contain benzocaine or lidocaine, which are used as a topical anesthetic.[1]

If the products are used as directed, they are fairly harmless. Most of these over-the-counter preparations however, end up in a diaper bag, easily accessible to an infant, toddler or young child, which presents a dangerous and potentially life-threatening situation. For example, if an older sibling comes across the little bottle or tube, and decides she wants to play mommy and give her baby brother his teething medicine, you now have a potential overdose on your hands. The older child might even ingest it.

According to Rose Ann Soloway, an administrator at the American Association of Poison Control Centers in Washington, D.C., ingestion of one of these topical anesthetics can cause strange, dangerous changes in the bloodstream. One teaspoon can change hemoglobin (a compound in red blood cells that transports oxygen to the bodily tissues), to methemoglobin, which can no longer carry oxygen to the cells. The essential deprivation of oxygen to all organs produces irregular heart rhythms, seizures, blue lips, blue nail beds and pale skin; essentially all organs are deprived of oxygen. Soloway states, "This is not a common situation, but it has happened."[2]

◆ *Toothpaste* ◆

There are basically three different types of toothpaste for a child: traditional toothpaste, a more naturally based one, and tooth powder. Most people don't think of toothpaste as being a potential health hazard for their children. In most cases it isn't, but there are those rare instances that need to be addressed. *(See chapter on "Fluoride.")*

Traditional Toothpaste

The more traditional toothpastes are usually made with abrasive substances (for polishing or bleaching), binders, anti-drying agents, detergent or foaming agents, flavoring agents, fluoride, sweeteners, coloring agents, water, preservatives and anti-plaque agents.[3]

Some of the ingredients fall into a questionable category. There are several different colors of food dye used to color toothpaste. According to one study published in *Pediatrics*, two of the more popular colors show adverse effects. FD&C blue #1 showed chromosomal damage and bronchoconstriction when combined with certain other colors. FD&C yellow #5 is responsible for a more extensive list of effects such as:

allergies, thyroid tumors, lymphocytic lymphomas, chromosomal damage, a trigger for asthma, urticaria (hives) and hyperactivity.[4]

Two of the more commonly used sweeteners in toothpaste are sorbitol and saccharin. According to a report by Winstron and Williams published in the *Journal of the American Dietetic Association,* "Sorbitol is a possible risk factor for diarrhea in young children." The report found that "Sorbitol malabsorption included gas, bloating, abdominal cramps and osmotic diarrhea." It also states that "7.5 grams of sorbitol, the amount in four pieces of sugar-free gum, four sugar-free breath mints, or one-and-a-half sugar-free lollipops, could cause diarrhea in a 3-year-old child."[5]

Saccharin, also known as the chemical 1, 2 benzisothiazolin-3-one-1, 1-dioxide (3), is an organic compound derived from petroleum, as well as a coal-tar derivative. It was removed from the "Generally Recognized as Safe" (GRAS) list in 1972 following a study released by the Wisconsin Alumni Research Foundation. The study suggested a possible link between saccharin and bladder cancer in rats.

Many studies on saccharin over the years show different findings, but despite the conflict, the Food and Drug Administration (FDA) proposed to ban the use of saccharin in April 1997. The public outcry for the non-caloric sweetener to remain on the market, however, was so strong, Congress passed the "Saccharin Study and Labeling Act" in November 1997, prohibiting the FDA from banning the substance pending further investigation. Congress has extended this moratorium seven times, the last one continuing through May 2002. The law brought with it a warning label for any product containing saccharin "Use of this product may be hazardous to your health. This product contains saccharin, which has been determined to cause cancer in laboratory animals."[6]

You will not, however, find this warning on a tube of toothpaste containing saccharin because it is not a food substance, but rather a hygiene product. The theory behind this is that the toothpaste is not being ingested so there should be no immediate health risk, unless of course your child decides to consume this sweetness. Frequently a tube of toothpaste is simply left on the bathroom counter making it very accessible for a child to reach.

Fluoride in toothpaste is another health risk that needs to be closely monitored. John Yiamouyiannis, author of *Fluoride: The Aging Factor*, describes the poisoning aspect of a child ingesting a 7-ounce or family size tube of toothpaste by quoting Proctor & Gamble, "theoretically at least, it contains enough fluoride to kill a small child."[7]

Natural Toothpastes & Powders

There are many natural toothpastes and powders on the market today. In most cases the ingredient lists are easy to read and thorough in describing each substance. Despite the more benign ingredients of the naturally based toothpastes, some of them still have fluoride, which in most cases is derived from naturally occurring ore, rather than a byproduct of aluminum or fertilizer companies. It is still however, considered to be a hazard if consumed in quantity. Adult supervision is again advised.

◆ Mouthwash ◆

Young children learn by imitation and mimic almost everything they see in one form or another. When they see Mom or Dad using mouthwash, even though the liquid is taken into the mouth and spit back out, a young mind will not always make the full connection. Children reflexively drink or swallow what goes into their mouths, especially if it looks like juice. So while they may drink the mouthwash like Mom and Dad, they don't usually spit it out like Mom and Dad.

Most mouthwash has more alcohol than beer, wine or hard liquor. They range in percentages, but some have as much as 30 percent alcohol, which equals an alcoholic beverage at 60 proof. Alcohol affects the central nervous system by producing a slower heart rate. Additionally, it lowers blood sugar levels, which can be dangerous in children because their systems haven't yet learned how to bring the levels back to normal. If blood sugar levels drop too low, it may result in seizures, coma or even death.[8]

• *Disclosing Tablets Or Solutions* •

Disclosing tablets are usually dispensed through school dental hygiene programs geared to teach children how to brush their teeth properly. The tablet is chewed, releasing dye into the mouth, or the liquid solution can be sipped from a cup and swished in the mouth, then spit out.

The red dye darkens the areas where the child has not brushed properly. This process shows them where they need to improve on brushing. Unfortunately, the tablets and solutions are made with FD&C Red #3 food dye (erythrosine), which, according to a study by the American Academy of Pediatrics Committee on Drugs, published in *Pediatrics*, October 1985, can cause adverse effects such as bronchoconstriction, sequential vascular response, elevation of protein-bound iodide, thyroid tumors, chromosomal damage and other unspecified symptoms.[9]

Even though the child is not supposed to ingest the product, there is always the possibility that some of the substance will be swallowed. Another consideration is the risk that the dye will be absorbed directly into the child's delicate system through the porous tissue of the mouth's cavity. Many parents have reported allergic reactions such as hyperactivity, upset stomachs, rashes, etc., after the use of products containing FD&C Red #3.[10]

It is wise to teach your child about the dangers of using red disclosing tablets or solutions that are loosely handed out in school education programs. Perhaps a discussion about the dangers of swallowing the substance, or its toxicity factor, will be enough to encourage the child not to participate in the event. The idea behind disclosing tablets is good, but their use could be hazardous to your child's health. Beet juice can be used in place of disclosing tablets or liquid solution. The result is not as strong in darkening the dirty area, but it still gives a good indication as to what spots will need more effort in brushing.

◆ Dental Sealants ◆

In the past 10 years, dental sealants have become a very popular technique to seal teeth against decay-causing bacteria. A thin plastic coating is painted primarily, but not exclusively, on the chewing surfaces of the back teeth.

Children get their first set of permanent molars somewhere between the ages of 5 and 7 years, and their second set between 11 and 14 years. The National Institute of Dental Research (NIDR) recommends that children get sealants on their permanent molars as soon as they come in.

Mothers & Others for a Livable Planet, Inc. a non-profit health and environmental advocacy group, published research on dental sealants in their newsletter, *The Green Guide*. Following are some key points of that research from Issue 30, October 1996:

Parents should beware: A study conducted by researchers at the University of Granada in Spain found that bisphenol-A (BPA) and a related substance bis-GMA, which are plastic chemicals used in dental sealants, behave much the same way as the female sex hormone estrogen.[11]

When the body is exposed to too much estrogen, especially in the form of synthetic or chemical-mimicking compounds, the delicate balance of the body can be thrown off. This chemical or substance is thus known as a hormone disruptor, which has the potential to disrupt endocrine or hormone function in the body. Estrogen is responsible for sending messages to the receiving genes. An overproduction of messages or messages sent at the wrong time, can affect reproductive organs in males and females, (i.e., the stimulation of breast cell growth, early puberty, fibroids, promotion of cancerous cell growth, and more), as well as behavior and other biological functions.[12]

In one clinical trial, college-aged volunteers were treated with one of four commercial dental resins based on BPA – Tetric, Charisma, Peralux and Delton. Their saliva was tested before and after the treatment. A significant amount of BPA, 3-30 micrograms per milliliter, was found in the saliva collected one hour after the application. Further studies are being done to determine how long the chemicals may continue to leak from the sealant.

BPA may stimulate human cells to grow in the same way estrogen does at levels lower than what was found in the saliva. Pregnant women should also be cautious of the dangerous effects that exposure to hormones and hormonelike chemicals could have on a developing fetus, such as reproductive disorders and some cancers.

Frederick vom Saal, Ph.D., of the University of Missouri, Columbia, is an expert on the effects of hormones. He thinks that there are a lot of unanswered questions about the long-term effects of dental sealants. While some dentists may recommend the sealants for baby teeth, vom Saal warns that the younger the individual, the more sense it makes to avoid exposure. He also says, "I would be concerned about the possibility of high levels of this chemical getting into a child. And until we learn more about its biological effects, as a parent I would therefore err on the side of caution."[13]

Other studies have been conducted to try and replicate the initial findings of the mimicking affects of BPA, but they have not seen the same results. Vom Saal believes this is because of the inadequate conditions under which the studies have been conducted. BPA can also be found in items such as tableware designed for children, teething rings, baby bottles and other plastic toys, depending on the manufacturer.[14]

BPA-based materials are also used in plastic resin composite fillings, but vom Saal says, "The amount released is a fraction of the surface area, and you are pinpointing a very small area in a filling as opposed to using the material to coat teeth."[15] In addition to BPA, another threat in certain sealants is Helioseal F, which is actually fluoride. This sealant is formulated as a time-released compound. It is hard to know exactly how much fluoride is being released and what effects it will have on a child's bones, organs and immune system. *(See chapter on "Fluoride.")*

• Plastic Teethers •

Certain plastic teething products can also cause problems for your child. *Consumer Reports* showed that government studies confirm that many teethers contain a chemical called di-isononyl-phthalate or DINP. Edward Groth, Ph.D., who oversaw the studies, states, "When babies chew on some plastics, they can leach a potentially harmful chemical called DINP. The soft plastics are made with polyvinyl chloride and contain DINP."[16]

According to *Consumer Reports*, May 1999, animal studies found that when consumed in high doses, DINP caused cancer, kidney damage, liver damage and other adverse affects. The report states, "Teethers are specifically designed to be 'mouthed' – and the chewing action can break down the plastic, accelerating the release of chemicals." The scientific community isn't sure whether it is harmful to children in the low levels they get from chewing on plastic objects, but feels that it makes sense to limit their exposure anyway. The government has asked manufacturers to reformulate their products, and most of them have cooperated.[17]

Since this is a new finding, it would be wise to throw away any teething device that may be in question. Look for the new package, which states that the teethers are free of the chemical DINP.

• Plastic Baby Bottles •

The Consumer Product Safety Commission also cautioned that DINP was not the only chemical that poses a problem to infant products. They found that when heated, plastic baby bottles made from polycarbonate, a clear and rigid plastic, a chemical called bisphenol-A was leached into infant formula. This is the same chemical that was discussed earlier, for its use in the composition of dental sealants. It also has estrogen-mimicking properties, which again, can interfere with normal development.[18]

According to *Consumer Reports*, based on testing done with an intact bottle, it was calculated that a baby who drank formula heated in a bottle made from polycarbonate would be exposed to a bisphenol-A dose of about 4 percent of the amount that had adversely affected test animals in studies.[19] Safety limits for exposure can be set as low as 0.1 percent of the level that has adversely affected animals. They state, "Babies who used the bottles tested could be exposed to a bisphenol-A dose forty times higher than that conservative definition of safety."[20]

Consumer Reports advice to parents is to dispose of polycarbonate baby bottles and replace them with bottles made of glass or polyethylene, an opaque, less-shiny plastic that does not leach bisphenol-A. To be sure the plastic bottles you are using are not made with bisphenol-A, contact the manufacturer and ask. The phone number should easily be found on the packaging.

◆ Amalgam (mercury or silver fillings) ◆

Many books have been written over the past 15 years examining the dangers of amalgam and mercury fillings. So many, in fact, that many European countries have stopped using mercury fillings in pregnant women and in children under 6 years old. Mercury can easily cross the placental barrier and be absorbed by the developing fetus. Frank Jerome D.D.S., author of *Tooth Truth* states, "The concentration of mercury may be higher in the embryo than in the mother." Mercury is a chemical known to cause birth defects and other reproductive harm.[21]

Is it possible that the mercury in "silver" dental fillings could play a part in building resistance to certain antibiotics? Yes, says microbiologist Anne Summers and her colleagues at the University of Georgia. They found that the mercury leached from amalgam can bring about changes in bacteria in the intestines, consequently developing resistance to commonly used antibiotics including penicillin, streptomycin and tetracycline.[22]

The first six weeks of pregnancy are crucial to a fetus. This is when all the basic organ systems are developing. If the mother is exposed to mercury, it is attracted to the embryo's developing central nervous system. The presence of these toxins can result in problems such as cleft palate, spina bifida or cerebral palsy.[23]

◆ General Anesthesia & Sedation ◆

When you choose a dentist for your child, it is important to investigate how much training the dentist has had in the area of general anesthesia. Medical anesthesiologists are required to have at least four years of anesthesia training after medical school. Unfortunately, many dentists and oral surgeons don't get this training, and some have as little as 60 hours.[24]

Working with children is different than working with adults. Children are much more susceptible in relation to their size and body weight to the effects of anesthesia and sedative drugs. According to Myron Yaster, pediatric anesthesiologist at John Hopkins Hospital, children need a deeper level of sedation and need to be monitored more closely. Yaster states, "When you take a child to that deeper level of sedation, you're on a slippery slope and it could very easily become catastrophic."[25]

You might ask, "How carefully are dentists being policed in regard to anesthesia or sedation drugs?" That depends on the individual dental boards of each state whose laws and enforcement vary. Interestingly enough, out of 52 states, only 32 state boards have the right to inspect dental offices. And according to an investigation by "60 Minutes II," of those 32, only 10 said they conduct regular inspections.

Peter Hartmann, a member of the California Dental Board states, "Since 1991, we've had a preponderance of child deaths in dental offices being caused by oral sedation." In California alone, over 200 children were injured from dental sedation or anesthesia between 1991-1999.[26]

Children as young as 3 years old have died as a result of sedation prior to a routine filling of a cavity. If your child needs to have a cavity filled, or any other dental work, and the dentist thinks it is in the best interest of the child to be sedated or have general anesthesia, do your homework. Investigate your dentist's qualifications before you consent to any kind of sedation.

Here are three important questions you may want to ask a dentist or oral surgeon:

1. What is your training in anesthesiology or conscious sedation? When in doubt, ask to see certification documents and check out their source.
2. What type of sedation will you be administering? If it is a combination of different drugs, educate yourself on the drug interactions.
3. Does your office have all the proper equipment for handling emergency

situations: i.e., pulse oximeter, IV equipment, a trach tube, EKG machine, crash cart, etc.?

Questions such as these can sometimes be intimidating to a dentist or doctor, but they could be instrumental in saving a child's life.

◆ *X-rays During Pregnancy* ◆

According to Lita Lee, Ph.D., author of *Radiation Protection Manual*, in 1958, Alice Stewart published the results of a large-scale epidemiological study finding that children whose mothers received X-rays during pregnancy had twice the risk of developing leukemia and other cancers before the age of 10. During the last months of pregnancy, the unborn child's rate of cancer risk doubles. If mom was X-rayed during her first trimester, the cancer risk was 10 times greater.[27] The formation of tooth buds begins in the first trimester of pregnancy, so it would stand to reason that X-rays taken during this time could adversely affect the developing teeth.

◆ *X-ray Exposure & Children* ◆

Since radiation in the body is cumulative, you should be extremely cautious about unnecessary X-rays. If your child does require an X-ray, make sure a lead shield is properly placed over the front of your child's chest, including the neck area where the thyroid gland is located.

When X-raying the mouth area there are three different formats – full mouth, where every tooth and all the roots are pictured; bitewing, where the top parts of the back teeth are pictured, allowing examination of surfaces between teeth and below the gum line; and periapical, which gives a good evaluation of the tips of the roots, the bone that surrounds the teeth and bone loss. X-rays should only be taken when necessary for specific evaluation. Repeated routine X-rays should be avoided.

Self-help:
According to Flora Parsa Stay, author of *The Complete Book of Dental Remedies*, beta-carotene is a good antioxidant and has preventive properties against cancerous cells. Calcium is also said to help protect against

radiation poisoning. Kelp is high in trace minerals, which bind with toxins that radiation causes and eliminates them. Vitamin C is known to promote the development of healthy tissue.[28]

Alfalfa and red clover are strong blood purifiers. And Stay also recommends the homeopathic remedy *Calcarea fluorica* to help prevent damage caused by extensive exposure to X-rays.[29]

✦ *Acidic Erosion of Tooth Enamel* ✦

Enamel erosion is most common with two types of children – those who love lemons and those who have a tendency towards vomiting. The thought of eating a lemon for most people stimulates a puckering of the lips, yet there are many children who crave them. Unfortunately, I have seen the teeth of some of these children just disintegrate. Over time, the acid in raw lemons has the potential to literally eat away the enamel.

If a child is prone to vomiting, the concern is that the stomach's hydrochloric acid can and will eventually erode the tooth enamel. It is important to pay special attention to the hygiene of these acidic teeth. This condition is common in children with reflex esophogitis, a hiatus hernia, or preteens and teens with eating disorders such as bulimia (these types of conditions allow stomach contents to seep into the mouth when lying down).[30]

✦ *Emergency Situations* ✦

Teeth ✦ *Broken* ✦ *Loose* ✦ *Knocked out*

Some estimates show that 50 percent of childhood injuries are related to teeth. If there is an injury to the mouth, stay calm. If there is bleeding, apply pressure until it stops. Clean the area gently with gauze or a washcloth soaked in 3% hydrogen peroxide, or a solution made with the mother tinctures of calendula and hypericum.

What you do for your child after an injury can make a big difference in saving a tooth or child's appearance and all around dental health. If a tooth has been hit or the child has fallen on it, close observation is a must. First, check for looseness. If there is inner bleeding the tooth will turn black. If there is any trauma to a tooth, do not use hot or cold directly in the mouth.[31]

If a permanent tooth becomes loose as a result of trauma, your dentist can rig a splint by attaching a wire to the tooth on either side to stabilize it, which will allow the gums and bones to heal. A baby tooth usually has the resiliency to heal on its own.

If a tooth breaks or is knocked out, remove it from the mouth immediately to prevent choking. If a baby tooth is knocked out, your biggest concern is probably the emotional trauma to the child. Barry Skaggs, D.D.S., a Beverly Hills oral and maxillofacial surgeon, suggests that if the tooth is literally hanging on by a thread to try to keep it in place by having the child bite lightly on a piece of gauze or tissue placed directly over the area, and get to an oral surgeon immediately.[32] If it is a permanent tooth and it is knocked out completely, time and procedure are of the utmost importance.

Approximately 5 million teeth are knocked out every year. A parent's response is crucial to successfully saving the child's tooth. When a tooth is knocked out it needs to be retrieved and protected for re-plantation into its socket. The root is extremely delicate, so it is important to hold the tooth by the crown or you may crush the tooth cells. Do not attempt to remove any debris off the tooth. The two primary causes of replanted tooth loss are tooth cell crushing and tooth cell dehydration. Once the tooth is knocked out, tooth cells begin to die within 15 minutes and within one to two hours enough cells will die that rejection of the tooth by the body is the usual outcome. Medical and dental research over the past 20 years has shown that the most effective storage system for preserving a tooth is with Hanks Balanced Salt Solution, a special pH balanced solution that will maintain normal cell metabolism (keeping cells alive) for longer periods of time.[33]

Paul Krasner, D.D.S., noted Professor of Endodontics at Temple University of Dentistry in Philadelphia, has developed the Save-A-Tooth preserving system. The Save-A-Tooth system uses a scientifically engineered removable basket and suspension net to protect the root system with Hanks

Balanced Salt Solution to preserve and reconstitute tooth cells. It is compact, portable and comes with a screw top and shatterproof container. Save-A-Tooth can be stored anywhere (emergency kit, car, daycare, etc.), does not need to be refrigerated, is inexpensive and has the American Dental Association Seal of Acceptance.

In 2003, the Ohio Department of Job and Family Services took the first step in leading our nation to healthier smiles by mandating all child-care facilities have first-aid items to save knocked-out teeth, and specifically recommends the Save-A-Tooth preserving system.[34]

According to Krasner, if the tooth is stored in his preserving system, even up to 24 hours, the cells still maintain their normal viability and there is a 90-percent success rate of re-plantation. The research using Hanks Balanced Salt Solution also shows that if a tooth is stored in these conditions for up to four days, there is still a 70-percent success rate. The council of Scientific Affairs of the American Medical Association, however, says the survival rate is highest if a dentist implants the tooth within one hour.[35]

Many dentists and professionals still don't know about Save-A-Tooth and recommend placing the tooth in milk to preserve it. While milk is better than nothing, it does not replace cell nutrients, which means the window of opportunity for a successful re-plantation narrows. Milk also needs to be refrigerated and, if sour, may cause tooth root cell damage. If you are using milk, or have no provisions for this rescue operation, time is of the essence. The best results are achieved if the tooth is implanted within the first 30 minutes of the accident. Despite all efforts, sometimes the pulp dies and a modified form of a root canal (pulpotomy) needs to be performed.[36]

Always contact your dentist or surgeon immediately for any medical emergency.

If a child's tooth is cracked or broken rather than knocked out, save any parts you can find and call your dentist. Fractures can range in severity and your dentist will be your best guide for determining your child's specific needs.

For a chip or shallow fracture, minor cosmetic or bonding repair may be all you need. Today's technology has developed composite plastic materials that can be molded, shaped and color-matched to the child's tooth. Deeper fractures may require immediate treatment to prevent infection or further complications. In severe cases a child may need a pulpotomy. Nerve damage may also occur as a result of trauma to a tooth. This can be tricky because nerve damage doesn't always show up right away and the dentist will need to check it every few months.[37]

If a baby tooth is lost before the permanent one moves into place, a space maintainer can be used to keep the other teeth from drifting. Be sure to discuss the situation with your dentist.

The dentist should also check for injuries to the jawbones, such as fractures or even dislocation. A trauma to the jaw can result in grave consequence if left untreated. The temporomandibular joint (TMJ) acts as a hinge between the upper and lower jawbones. If this area is injured it can affect the child's bite. For any type of trauma to the head there is always the option of consulting with a chiropractor trained in craniosacral therapy, in addition to your dentist.

Skaggs feels that if the injury to the jaw is a fracture, stabilization can usually be obtained through the use of an acrylic brace, which still allows movement of the mouth. An injury of this nature should heal in two or three weeks. Iced applications every few hours will also ease the injury by reducing inflammation and swelling, along with the homeopathic remedies *Arnica* and *Calcarea phosphorica*. The child may have to eat soft foods for a few weeks during the healing process.

If a tooth is pushed out of position, wait until the pain has stopped before applying gentle pressure to move it back to the original place. The tooth can be softly manipulated by using the thumb and index finger. Again notify the dentist of the situation because sometimes a serious trauma to a tooth can cause infection or damage to a developing tooth.

In some cases, a child will fall on a milk tooth causing it to recede back into the gum. This is called an intrusion and can sometimes affect the growing permanent tooth underneath. Depending on the severity of the fall, the eruption of the permanent tooth in rare cases may be delayed, stopped, malformed or even divided into a dilacerated or twin tooth. In most cases however, the tooth will eventually push back out on its own with no problems.[38]

Self-help:
1. Stay calm.
2. Knocked out tooth: depending on the age – remove tooth to prevent choking. Place the tooth in either Save-A-Tooth solution or milk to preserve it.
3. Injury with bleeding: apply pressure until bleeding stops or help can arrive. Gently clean the area with a sterile gauze or clean washcloth. A rinse of 3% hydrogen peroxide or the mother tinctures of calendula (works as an antiseptic) and hypericum or St John's wort (which is used to help relieve any nerve pain) can be used to help prevent infection. Contact a dentist or physician immediately.

The most common homeopathic remedies used for emergency teeth situations are:

Aconitum napellus – There is fear from the trauma.
Arnica montana – This remedy is for any trauma to the tissue or tooth. It reabsorbs the blood into the tissue, reduces inflammation and helps control bleeding.
Calcarea phosphorica – This remedy will help knit the bone or fracture back together.
Hypericum – This will help if there is any nerve involvement from the trauma.
Hepar sulphuris – There is an infection and the area is tender to the touch and the child is irritable.
Mercurius solubilis – An infection when there is a lot of saliva and the child is not very grouchy.

◆ Lost Fillings ◆

If a filling falls out, there are a few things you can do to ease discomfort and to help prevent infection until you can contact your dentist (always call for an emergency consultation).

Self-help:
Oil of clove* is a great nerve sedative, as well as an anesthetic to relieve pain. The clove oil can be mixed with a little olive oil, so that it isn't too hot for the child. Always test the mixture on your own gums to find the right blend. Dip a piece of cotton or gauze in the oil and dab or drip it onto the area. A toothpick with a small piece of cotton wrapped on the end can be a good precision tool for the situation.

The mother tincture of *Plantago major* is another effective topical remedy for toothache pain, especially pain that radiates between teeth, ears and the sinus canal.

There is also a temporary filling substance called DenTemp. This material will help seal off the area from food and air temporarily until you can get to the dentist. The one drawback to using this product is, if the tooth is abscessed, pressure can build underneath and may cause even more pain to the child. If this does happen, remove the temporary filling immediately.

◆ Toothache ◆

There are several reasons why a child experiences a toothache – an abscess in the gum or root, a deep cavity into the nerve area, teeth crowding, or a crack or break in a tooth. Another possibility is when children are under a lot of stress or going through hormonal changes, sometimes their teeth become sensitive to temperatures or touch.

Self-help:
The most common homeopathic remedies for a toothache are:

Aconitum napellus – A child is frantic with pain and fear; a hot face; the symptoms come on suddenly, perhaps after exposure to a cold drink or wind.
Belladonna – A cutting pain in the root of the tooth especially on biting down; flushed face; hot, delirious, throbbing pain, which is better from

pressure.

Chamomilla – The child is irritable with extreme pain; wants things, then doesn't want them; one cheek may be red and the other pale.

Hepar sulphuris – An infection is present; the child is grumpy and the area is sensitive to touch.

Hypericum – Pain in the nerve that shoots suddenly like a lightning bolt.

Mercurius solubilis – A toothache due to infection with a lot of saliva and a metallic taste in the mouth.

Silicea – There is an infection with a lot of sweating and bad breath.

◆ Correctional Appliances ◆

If your orthodontic or correctional appliance breaks or bends, be sure to contact your doctor immediately. If there are any sharp wires, orthodontic wax can be applied to the wire to protect the inside of the mouth from being cut.

◆ Tongue ◆ Cheek ◆ Cuts ◆

If your child bites his tongue or cheek, or has a cut in his mouth that is bleeding, apply pressure to the area with gauze. You can also ice the area, but be careful not to put the ice directly on the skin as it can attach and get stuck, pulling layers of skin off with it. This can be extremely painful. Put the ice in a moistened washcloth or gauze before applying it to the area. Cuts or lacerations in the mouth should be treated in much the same way to stop bleeding, providing there is no other foreign object or splinter in the wound. Always have a professional assess the situation immediately.

◆ Burns ◆

Burns of the mouth are common to children. In some cases a burn can be quite serious and may require medical attention. If your child burns his mouth you can immediately flush the mouth with cool water. One of the most effective burn remedies I have ever come across is called "Willard's Water XXX."

Willard's Water was formulated and patented by the late John Willard, Sr.,

Professor Emeritus of Chemistry at the South Dakota School of Mines and Technology. It is Catalyst Altered Water, which promotes first generation healing (healing from the inside out, rather than the outside in).

The ratio you use to mix Willard's Water is very important. Directions on the
label state, "Mix two ounces of Willard's Water XXX concentrate to one gallon of distilled water." I always have a gallon of the mixture prepared for any emergency burn situations. Once diluted the mixture should be stored in the refrigerator. I also keep a few ounces in a spray bottle.

For minor burns of the tongue or lips, use the spray bottle. Spray the area repeatedly until the pain is gone (usually for a few minutes). For more severe burns on the roof of the mouth sip a cup of the water and hold it in the mouth for as long as possible (Willard's Water is non-toxic and according to the company safe to ingest), repeating the process over and over until there's no more pain and/or blister.

Self-help:
Caution: Never apply ointments, salves, butter or ice to a burn. Never break the blisters. In case of severe burns, seek professional medical attention immediately.
1. Flush area with cool water.
2. Always have Willard's Water on hand. It can be used both topically and internally to help replenish fluids, and takes away pain almost instantly.
3. *Five Flower* or *Rescue Remedy* can be used externally on the wrist to help calm the child down so appropriate measures can be taken to help.

The most common homeopathic remedies used for burns of the mouth are:

Arnica Montana – There is severe trauma to the skin and shock.
Cantharis – This is usually the first remedy given for burns.
Phosphorus – Used for electrical burns.
Urtica urens – If the burn continues to sting for a long time.

Conclusion

I encourage parents to educate themselves in all of these areas of importance - cautions, hazards and emergency situations and to always use common sense. Knowledge is power and this wisdom could be instrumental in saving a tooth or even a life of an innocent child.

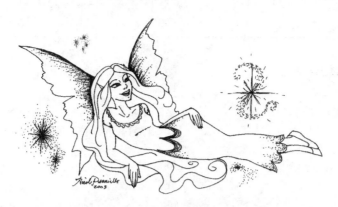

"The tooth fairy has been around since the beginning of recorded time. She's a full-fledged, card-carrying fairy and her best friends are all fairies, angels and God. She lives in Heaven, but she travels almost all the time. She loves things that are white and that sparkle, so she's really happy when kids do a good job keeping their teeth clean.

I bet you've always wondered where the tooth fairy takes teeth. Well, she takes them to a very special large room in Heaven. This room is the Wish Room. These beautiful sparkling white gems line the walls in the room where the fairies make wishes come true. The tooth fairy gives money to help the kids realize how precious their teeth are.

The tooth fairy travels in a most unique way. First, she's given a list of kids to visit. Then, all she has to do is focus on one of the names and like magic, she appears in their bedroom to make the exchange. She has to be very quiet so she doesn't wake the tooth-giving child, or any brothers and sisters who might be sleeping in the same room.

She has long, blond, curly hair that glistens when the light shines on it – kind of like it has tiny jewels everywhere. She always wears white and her outfits flow in the soft summer breeze. She has wings that are smaller than angel wings and are made of a light lavender shimmering material. She wears a white velvet pouch which is where she puts the teeth she collects every night.

I'm so happy that there is a tooth fairy and I'm so happy that my teeth have helped cover the walls of her special Wish Room. Take good care of your teeth and she will be back to your house very soon."

Dea – A mother's fable

Chapter Eight

Keeping Teeth Clean

◆ Teeth Brushing & Oral Hygiene ◆

To a child or teen, the care of teeth can seem inconsequential. But as adults, we know the advantages and disadvantages of taking care of our teeth. The result of poor hygiene habits can and will influence us for the rest of our lives. That is why teaching our children responsible dental care is essential.

The best way to educate a child about the care of teeth is to be a good role model and brush regularly. Approaching our own dental care with a positive attitude will teach them to do the same. Children should know that good hygiene today would influence the health of their adult teeth tomorrow.

◆ The Early Years ◆

A good time to start taking care of teeth is long before there are any visible signs of them. Rubbing or massaging a child's gums once or twice a day with a clean finger or piece of gauze will help stimulate gum circulation, and promote healthy gums and teeth. When the first tooth arrives, wiping it off with a clean gauze cloth after each feeding will help keep bacteria levels down.

Once the child starts walking, invite them to join you whenever you are going to brush your teeth (hopefully after every meal). They will usually start to show an interest in a toothbrush somewhere between the age of 18 months and 2 years. Each child responds differently to this exercise – some gladly participate and others have no interest. If you make something look fun, children usually want to be involved. Be patient – eventually they will take you up on the offer.

◆ Choosing The Right Toothbrush ◆

A child's first toothbrush should be small with soft bristles, unless otherwise recommended by your dentist. There is a wide selection of toothbrushes on the market today. They come in many shapes and sizes. The main features to look for are: Bristles – well-rounded, so as not to injure gum tissue; they should be welded or fused, not stapled. Studies show that welding offers a cleaner hygienic environment over the stapled/clamped process by reducing the opportunity for harmful anaerobic bacteria to multiply[1]; Handle – it should feel comfortable; Head size - age appropriate. As the child grows, so does his need for a larger brush. In most cases, the use of soft bristles is still preferred.

◆ Alternative Toothbrushes ◆

Toothbrushes that are environmentally conscious and made from 100 percent recyclable materials are always preferable. Some even come with interchangeable heads. Recently at the Natural Products Expo West in Anaheim, I saw a large display container of discarded toothbrushes, which took up quite a bit of space. Right next to that display was another container filled with just the heads, taking up a fraction of the space, effectively illustrating the environmental impact of toothbrushes, especially since toothbrushes should be replaced every three months. Anything we can do to help reduce waste in our environment is a plus.

One company that has jumped on the bandwagon for the environment is called Recycline, offering a Preserve Jr. brush. It doesn't have interchangeable heads, but it is made of recycled plastic and is 100 percent recyclable into other cool products. The brush comes with a postage-paid recycling mailer to send your used brush back to the company.

Another environmentally friendly toothbrush that has an interchangeable head is the Terradent-Fun Brush distributed by Eco-Dent International. It has rounded bristles welded to the head, a flexible neck that distributes brushing pressure, to protect gum tissue, and is designed to encourage proper gripping instruction for a young brusher.

According to Marc Warsowe, president of Eco-Dent International, "In tests conducted by Oko-Test, a leading German consumer magazine, Terradent toothbrushes scored higher than any other brand – including Oral-B, Colgate, Sensodyne, Dr. Best (Aquafresh), and Fuchs in 'head-to-head' quality competitions."[2]

The Fuchs toothbrush made by Ekotec also has interchangeable heads, but it only comes in a standard size that is more suitable for older children. Fuchs does, however, have a child's junior-size brush with a stationary head, which has rounded and polished bristles and a stylized gripping handle for better coordination.

The Collis Curve toothbrush, developed by George C. Collis, D.D.S., is an unusual brush that deserves mention. The brush has two outer rows of soft curved bristles that surround a center row of short straight bristles. This toothbrush cleans all surfaces of the tooth at once. Dr. Collis invented the toothbrush for his elderly father who was no longer able to care for his own teeth. Collis needed a device that was efficient in its hygiene ability, and easy for a caregiver to maneuver in hard-to-reach places.

Collis found that his toothbrush was not only perfect for the elderly, but also for children, including those with special needs. Collis states, "The design minimizes position changes needed for effective brushing and improves ease of access to more obscured dental surfaces."[3]

The Collis Curve is a funny looking toothbrush, but in studies against a manual conventional toothbrush it was found to be more effective in the removal of plaque, and equally as effective as the electric Interplak.[4,5] The Collis also significantly improved the condition of the gingiva when used by middle-school children in grades six, seven and eight.[6]

The Baby Collis Curve brush is ideal for baby's first toothbrush (after 2 years of age the company recommends its Junior brush).

Although their toothbrushes have no environmentally conscious benefit, Oral-B has developed a series of toothbrushes for the different stages of childhood: Stage one (4 to 24 months) addresses sensitive gums with baby-soft bristles for massaging gums and cleaning baby's first teeth; stage two (2 to 4 years) is designed for smaller hands that have limited dexterity with a narrow brushhead and a power tip to reach back teeth; stage three (5 to 7 years) has a power tip and cup-shaped bristles to surround and clean teeth as the primary ones start falling out; stage four (8 years and older) has varying bristle textures and levels to better maneuver around the gaps and holes of missing teeth and tender gums of older children. All stages have a cushioned head that protects gums from irritation.

No toothbrush section would be complete without discussing the all time fun hygiene toy, an electric toothbrush. In April 1997, the *Journal of the American Dental Association (JADA)* reported on the first investigation in 20 years of children and use of an electric toothbrush. The Braun Oral-B Plaque Remover for Kids was the electric toothbrush used in this study. The study involved children 8 to 12 years of age. Examiners found significantly greater plaque removal in children who used the electric toothbrush vs. a manual brush.[7] The authors state, "This finding is consistent with the hypothesis that electric toothbrushes can overcome the need for good brushing technique and manual dexterity." The researchers feel that if nothing else, the brush itself is a motivation tool for a child to brush more often.[8] A young child should always be supervised when using an electric toothbrush.

Other studies confirm the efficiency of certain power toothbrushes vs. manual toothbrushes in improving oral health of adolescents wearing orthodontic appliances. In 1984, Pro-Dentec, one of the earlier companies to produce an electric toothbrush, released its Rota-Dent brush. A 1989 study compared the Rota-Dent, which is only available through dental offices, with a conventional toothbrush. The 18-month evaluation concluded that the rotary electric toothbrush was more effective in maintaining good periodontal health during fixed orthodontic treatment. [9]

In 1996, 40 adolescent patients were found to have a 20-percent reduction of plaque at a 12-week evaluation with overall improved gingival health.[10]

Then in 1997, 24 11- to 18-year-olds experienced a threefold plaque reduction with a 69-percent improvement of gingival bleeding.[11] The Sonicare sonic-powered toothbrush was used against a manual toothbrush in both of these later studies.

No matter which brush you end up purchasing, the maintenance is the same. It is important to rinse the toothbrush thoroughly after each use because the moist environment tends to harbor bacteria. If the child has any type of infection of the gums, throat, mouth, cold or flu, viral or bacterial, disinfect the brush by soaking it in hydrogen peroxide or a citricidal solution (grapefruit seed extract) to help eliminate recurrent or further infection, or consider a replacement.[12]

Ideally a toothbrush (head) should be replaced every three months. If the bristles are showing signs of wear and tear, such as being frayed, flat or bent prior to this time, it would be prudent to make the change sooner. A brush in a compromised condition can injure or irritate gum tissue and is not capable of cleaning teeth properly.

◆ *Brushing & Technique* ◆

All you really need to get started is water and a toothbrush. In fact, when you first introduce the toothbrush to your child it will generally be used as a chewing instrument. Slowly, the child will become familiar with the brush and its function, offering you an opportunity to give gentle guidance about which way the bristles need to face, etc.

Experts agree the key components to good oral hygiene are technique and manual dexterity. Some people brush their teeth hard and rough and consider this a good technique. But it isn't how hard you brush that counts, it is how thoroughly you brush.

According to one German dentist, the technique in learning to brush properly advances with different stages of development. Between the ages of 2 and 4 years old, a child brushes with straight movements, giving only the ability to effectively clean the chewing surfaces of the teeth. By the age of 4, most children are capable of drawing a big circle, which is the movement needed to clean the outer surfaces of their teeth. When a child starts school and learns to write, they begin to train their fine motor (movement) skills and develop the coordination necessary to draw little circles for cleaning a tooth's inner surface.[13] As their coordination improves, so will their technique. One English study in 1978 showed that children at 5 years of age only clean about 25 percent of the tooth surface. By age 11, they manage to clean about half, and as young adults 67 percent.[14]

Be creative with your approach. The practice of brushing, rinsing and spitting can be a lot of fun for kids. Most children love to play games so you may want to start by encouraging them to feel the brush tickle their gums and teeth. This game should be played long before toothpaste enters into the equation. Eventually, your child will perfect their method and then it will be time to add toothpaste; Weleda makes a gentle enzyme tooth gel excellent for beginners, made with natural ingredients. *(See resources in back of book.)*

Begin with a very small amount of toothpaste - less than the size of a small pea. According to Thomas McGuire, D.D.S., author of *Tooth Fitness*, this is very important because most children between the ages of 2 and 6 years swallow about one-third of the toothpaste used during a brushing. This decreases to 20 percent between the ages of 7 and 16. If toothpaste contains ingredients such as fluoride, chemicals, sweeteners or dyes, its use should be closely monitored as it can pose a health risk to children. Children are more susceptible to toxic levels and poisonings because of their size and body weight.[15] *(See the chapter on "Hazards, Cautions & Emergency Situations.")*

A parent should give daily brushing guidance to a young child. As they get older, parents should review the child's technique often and continue to give positive encouragement. Technique is not something you are born with; it is something that is taught. But because most of us have never been taught technique, we don't know how to teach it.

Most dentists suggest the same thing, follow a specific pattern and rhythm, be consistent. It's best to choose one side and start at the very back, working your way around to the other side. Start with the outside surfaces of the lower teeth, then proceed to the upper teeth. (It doesn't really matter which side or surface you start with, just be consistent.) Continue with the same format on the inside surfaces. Work hard to get those back teeth because most often they don't get the same attention as the front ones. It's important to finish the process by brushing all chewing surfaces.

Both frequency and efficiency are the key to healthy teeth. Once children have mastered the basic technique, they are ready to learn proper positioning and motion of the brush. Place the bristles gently against the gum line, massaging the gum tissue, and then rolling it in the direction in which the teeth grow.

When you are done brushing all teeth, be sure to brush the tongue. The tongue is also a gracious host to bacteria. Studies show that the tongue is a major source of oral debris and plaque. By simply cleaning the tongue, you can reduce oral debris and retard the total plaque accumulation on the teeth.[16,17]

There are several ways to clean a tongue: 1) with a toothbrush: brushing the tongue from back to front, rinsing the brush after each stroke; 2) a tongue cleaner: plastic or stainless steel (probably for the older child), instructions with purchase; 3) or a small spoon: place the concave side down and drag it lightly from back to front, again rinsing after each stroke. Keep in mind that tongue cleaning may trigger a gag reflex in children so start by cleaning small sections from the middle forward.

Many dentists suggest brushing three times a day for three minutes. Unfortunately, this is an unrealistic goal for most adults let alone young children. One minute, two times a day in the beginning is more realistic. For school-aged children, increase the time as patience dictates, again at least two times a day. You will get more brushing time out of your child if she is sitting down. For some children, listening to stories will help distract them from the amount of time they are putting into the event. Experiment with what works best for your family.

The best times for brushing are in the morning and just before bedtime. Plaque forms while you sleep because there is less production of saliva during this time, especially if the child is a mouth breather. If this plaque is not removed in the morning, it will give the bacteria a chance to breed on the teeth all day. Nighttime brushing is essential to cleanse the mouth of all debris and bacteria that has accumulated over the course of the day.

Some dentists encourage dry brushing occasionally, because it may be more effective in helping dislodge plaque. Be sure to check with your dentist to determine your child's individual needs.

It is much easier to inspire good brushing habits now rather than having to restrain or anesthetize your child for restorative dentistry later. Negative feelings about early dental experiences may set the stage for long-term anxiety about dental care.

◆ *Flossing & Water Irrigation Systems* ◆

No matter how well you think you have brushed, there is always more debris lurking in those cracks and crevices that flossing and water picking can help eliminate.

Flossing is an important aid to reaching those hard-to-clean spots. Most often, flossing is recommended for children with teeth that are crowded or touching. Food tends to get stuck in these crevices and cause decay. Some dentists suggest flossing before you brush, while others prefer after – it comes down to personal preference.

Technique is also required in the use of dental floss. To clean in between the teeth, gently and slowly move the floss in an up-and-down and back-and-forth motion. If you have reservations, ask your dentist to demonstrate proper flossing methods.

To clean the gums, curve the floss around the base of the tooth. Gently move the floss back and forth under the gums. When removing the floss, use the same motions. Avoid snapping the floss; which can injure the gum tissue. Waxed dental floss is gentler on the gum tissue.

Eco-Dent International offers its alternative to dental floss, Gentle Floss.

They were one of the first floss manufacturers to use natural enzymes for its anti-bacterial properties, and is made with a blend of 100 percent plant waxes and essential oils.

Tom's of Maine also has a flossing ribbon similar to dental floss. The floss comes in either a flat or round nylon ribbon, which is coated with a unique combination of natural waxes and flavored with pure mint oils. Nature's Gate has also come out with natural floss in three flavors, Tea Tree, mint and anise, all soaked in green tea for it's antibacterial and antioxidant properties. If you are ready to try a more natural type of floss, then give one of these a try. All three companies take pride in their environmentally friendly packaging.

Water irrigation machines are another effective means for removing pieces of debris in those hard-to-reach places and stimulating gum circulation. Always use a water system on the lowest setting for children unless otherwise specified by your dentist or orthodontist. The pressure from higher settings can push particles up under the gum line. If not used properly a water irrigation system may cause damage to gum tissue or even contribute to infection.

♦ *Natural Toothpaste* ♦

Over the years, the toothpaste industry has grown into a multibillion-dollar-a-year business. While most commercial toothpastes are inviting to consumers through big advertising campaigns, they can be misleading when it comes to good health.

There are so many different brands of children's toothpaste on the market today it can be difficult to choose the best one for your family. For the most part, people are not educated about the ingredients found in toothpaste or what their functions are. Most commercial toothpastes have synthetic ingredients such as artificial sweeteners, colors (dyes) and flavorings, chemical preservatives and detergents. An ingredient comparison gives a clearer picture.

Crest Regular Flavor Toothpaste
(a commercial toothpaste)

Sodium fluoride: prevents tooth decay; toxic in large doses • Sorbitol: a binder, sweetener, and humectant • water: for consistency • hydrated silica: a dioxide of the glassy mineral silicon combined with water; an abrasive and anti-caking agent • trisodium phosphate: a synthetic emulsifier and texturizer • sodium lauryl sulfate: a surfactant and emulsifier • flavor: usually synthetic when unspecified • sodium phosphate: a buffering agent • xanthan gum: a thickener, emulsifier, and stabilizer; produced by carbohydrate fermentation • carbomer 956: a synthetic thickener and emulsifier • sodium saccharin: an artificial sweetener that has been shown to cause cancer in laboratory animals • titanium dioxide: a silver-colored metallic chemical element used as white coloring • FD&C Blue #1: a coal tar derivative coloring agent; has caused tumors in laboratory animals.

Nature's Gate – Cherry flavor
(a natural based toothpaste)

Free calcium: a calcium ion derived from carrots; strengthens teeth and helps protect tooth enamel • vegetable glycerin: maintains freshness; as a natural humectant, acts to protect and soothe gums • silica: mild abrasive; cleans and polishes; helps remove plaque • purified water: free of spores, impurities and hard minerals; maintains freshness • hydrogenated starch hydrolysate: a natural sweetener obtained by reduction of a special high maltose syrup • goldenseal: has antiseptic properties • methylparaben: a bactericide derived from gum benzoin • cellulose gum: derived from plant fibers; a thickener and stabilizer • sodium lauryl sulfate: a mild foaming cleanser derived from coconut oil • natural flavors: pure cherry extract • calcium ascorbate: a form of vitamin C • natural colors: annatto and carmine.

If you introduce your child to natural toothpaste from the start, it will teach them about smart hygiene and good health practices at an early age. Fortunately there are many natural products available today that taste good. The most popular ones for kids are: Nature's Gate – cherry or mint gel or anise; Jason – peppermint, deep sea spearmint, citrus and spice; The

Natural Dentist – bubble gum or spicy cinnamon; Weleda – children's (gentle enzyme) tooth gel, mint and other flavors; Tom's of Maine – strawberry, orange, cinnamint, and mint; Boiron – anise or lemon. These toothpastes have no sugar, dyes, synthetic chemicals or artificial sweeteners.

Regardless of what toothpaste you choose, look for a gentle formula. When toothpaste is too harsh or abrasive, it erodes the tooth's enamel (top layer) over time. Enamel has a white appearance and protects teeth. Once this layer is gone, not only does a tooth become more susceptible to problems, it exposes the under layer, called dentin, which is more yellow in color.

The Natural Dentist and certain flavors of Tom's of Maine toothpaste contain a natural form of fluoride. The companies state that their fluoride comes from calcium fluoride, a naturally occurring mined ore. Fluorine is a trace mineral found in soil, fresh water and salt water, as well as in several foods. Even though the fluoride in these toothpastes are from a natural source, caution should still be exercised as fluoride (natural or not), if consumed in large quantities, may still be hazardous. Adult supervision is always advised.[18]

Results from several studies comparing the benefits of natural and regular toothpastes show that natural brands like the Natural Dentist's Herbal Toothpaste and Gum Therapy produced the largest zones of inhibition against three types of bacteria when up against: Cool Mint Listerine, Crest Gum Care, Crest Regular and Colgate Regular.[19] And when studied against Colgate Total, they were significantly better in maintaining reductions in plaque and stain that were obtained after the initial baseline cleaning was compared.[20]

◆ *Tooth powder* ◆

Eco-Dent tooth powder is a natural powder made with mineral salts, baking soda, and natural flavoring oils. The powder has what the company calls a "unique effervescent action" which it claims is not possible with tube type pastes. Effervescent action is "the chemical reaction that generates carbon dioxide (CO_2) gas when an acid and a base are combined." This action manifests when water and a toothbrush touch the powder, producing a bubbling and fizzing action. Independent and unsponsored research conducted at major universities in the United States and Europe showed that when the extra CO_2 mixes with saliva it creates additional carbonic acid, which in turn creates more mineral ions that enhance natural remineralization.[21]

Remineralization can be defined as the replacement of the minerals in the teeth that were lost as a result of a cariogenic (acid) challenge. Eco-Dent explains that certain conditions must occur simultaneously in order to create this remineralization process: a higher concentration of carbonic acid; an environment supercharged with all minerals needed for remineralizing the teeth (including trace minerals, present in natural sea salt); and a clean surface (created by the foaming action), to allow the remineralizing ions exposure to the demineralized enamel.

The independent studies found Eco-Dent helped strengthen and harden dental enamel using minerals in the mouth, achieving a superior net remineralization when compared to Colgate with MFP Fluoride. It also showed a better performance in preventing decay-causing oral bacteria from binding to teeth and was also less abrasive.[22]

◆ *Mouthwash* ◆

Many mouthwash manufacturers claim their products kill germs and offer fresh breath. What they don't tell you is that conventional mouthwashes may contain as much as 30 percent alcohol to kill these germs. Numerous studies have linked high alcohol content to oral cancer. These commercial brands may present a poisoning hazard to small children.[23] *(See chapter on "Hazards, Cautions, & Emergency Situations.')*

With the size of the natural products industry today, there are equally beneficial and tasty mouthwashes available without alcohol, dyes, chemicals, synthetic preservatives, sugar, artificial sweeteners, flavors or fragrances.

Instead, natural manufacturers offer healing and soothing herbs such as echinacea and goldenseal, which have been known to kill the germs that cause gingivitis as effectively as those with alcohol (without the added risk of cancer.) Some of the other herbs include calendula, an anti-inflammatory agent, aloe, chamomile, and bloodroot. Additional ingredients found in some natural mouthwashes include vitamin C, the antioxidant CoQ10, grapefruit seed extract and essential oils (sage, clove, eucalyptus, geranium, mints, and cinnamon) for flavoring as well as their healing properties.[24]

The most popular natural brands for children are: The Natural Dentist – cherry, mint or spicy cinnamon; Eco-Dent – tangy orange-clove, spicy cool cinnamon or mint; Tom's of Maine – spearmint, cinnamint, peppermint baking soda or gingermint baking soda flavors; Peelu – cinnamon or mint.

One study conducted at the New York University College of Dentistry showed that The Natural Dentist's Herbal Mouth and Gum Therapy produced larger zones of microbial inhibition than Listerine and Scope against three different bacteria tested. The Mouth and Gum Therapy also showed larger zones of microbial inhibition than the prescription mouthwash Peridex on two of the three bacteria tested, and produced similar zones of inhibition against the third bacteria. In another study, at the same university, it was proven to help reduce gingivitis and gingival bleeding.[25]

♦ *Dental Chewing Gum* ♦

Chewing sugarless dental gum is an easy way to address oral hygiene for kids on the go. Several companies have come up with a natural dental chewing gum as a quick fix for dirty teeth. This is definitely not the preferred method for teeth cleaning and healthy gums, but when you are in a situation where brushing is difficult, dental chewing gum offers another option.

The Peelu Dental Chewing Gum contains natural fibers from the peelu tree (*Salvadora persica*) found in Asia, Africa and the Middle East. Its name means, "Tree for Tooth Care," and in some countries they refer to it as "the toothbrush tree."

In three scientific studies (Rostock University, Dhahrans University, Indiana University) it was found that peelu fibers contain a natural chlorine with whitening abilities to remove tarter and stains. In addition, the researchers established that peelu resins form a coating over the enamel to help protect teeth from decay.[26]

The makers of Peelu Dental Chewing Gum also make a toothpaste and powder, and in April 1991, were granted a patent for the only dental care product to use a plant fiber as its cleansing agent. (You didn't see the toothpaste and powder mentioned in the sections on tooth powder or paste, as they have a strange consistency and taste that take some getting used to and are not kid friendly, but the gum tastes great.)[27] The gum is available in four flavors: peppermint, spearmint, cinnamon and mixed fruit.

Eco-Dent International also offers a chewing gum, Between! Dental Gum, with all the dental health benefits of natural baking soda, minerals, antioxidants (A, C and E at 25 percent daily value), slippery elm, stevia and xylitol.[28] The company offers this gum in cool mint, cinnamon and wintergreen flavors.

There is enough clinical evidence regarding the effectiveness of xylitol against caries for gum manufacturers to take notice. One study conducted in Belize, involving 1,277 school children, aged 9 and 10 years old, confirmed the effectiveness of xylitol in reducing the risk of dental caries. Children chewing a gum containing xylitol five times a day showed a 70-percent lower caries risk than the group that didn't chew gum. (I personally don't promote the chewing of gum five times a day), and a 50-percent lower risk of cavities, than the group chewing gum containing just Sorbitol. Those chewing sucrose (sugar) gum on a regular basis appeared to experience no benefit in preventing dental caries.[29]

Another relatively new ingredient to the public's eye is *Stevia rebaudiana*. Stevia is a South American herb found in Paraguay, Uruguay, and Central America, and has been used by natives for hundreds of years. The leaves of this shrub are the sweetest natural product known to date (much sweeter than sugar). It produces no calories, won't raise blood sugar levels or cause tooth decay. Studies show that stevioside (one of the main compounds of the stevia leaf, a pure white crystalline extract) can inhibit the growth of microbes such as *Streptococcus mutans, Lactobacillus plantarum* and *Lactobacillus casei*. Stevia's ability to retard the growth of plaque in the mouth and help reduce cavities makes it a positive addition to dental products (dental gum, mouthwashes, toothpastes, etc.).[30,31] Stevia is also a perfect alternative to sugar, cane juice, or synthetic sweeteners for baking or sweetening herbal tea. *(See resources in back of book.)*

Conclusion

There are many healthy products that taste good and are effective in maintaining optimum oral health. With all of the choices available, we can begin to develop a dental hygiene plan for the family that works for everyone. When children and parents come together to prevent tooth decay, make visiting the dentist a pleasant experience and support companies that continually provide cost effective, recyclable, responsible and healthy products, we all win.

"When our daughter Selina lost her first tooth, I'm not sure who was more excited, her or us. I remember her tooth was barely hanging on and we just kept tugging and pulling on it. Her father and I were torn about what to put under her pillow that night in exchange for the tooth. Money seemed so superficial, so we decided to give her a sun catcher to fill her room with rainbow fairies every morning. She was so excited the next morning and loved what the tooth fairy had given her."

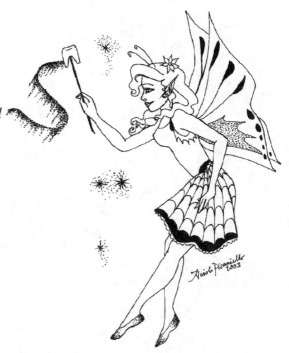

Laura – A mother's thoughts

"Well, I think she is a good princess who lives in a castle made of children's teeth that have already fallen out. She watches over them. She also sprinkles dust on them when their teeth fall out to make sure that their grown-up teeth come in the way they're supposed to, but I don't know for sure and she hasn't come to visit me yet!"

Hannah – 5 years old

"When I was in kindergarten, I sat down for lunch next to two boys. The boys dared me to yank out my loose tooth – so I did and that tooth is my best now. As for the tooth fairy, one day I demanded that my mom tell me if the tooth fairy was real. She told me that it was fake and I felt much more comfortable."

Samantha – 9 years old

Chapter Nine

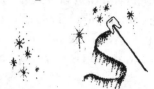

Correcting Crooked Teeth

◆ How to Correct Crooked Teeth ◆

In order to fully understand how the process of correcting teeth works, it is important to have a general knowledge of the anatomy and mechanics of the head or skull.

◆ Anatomy Of The Jaw ◆

The mouth is actually an organ called the oral cavity. The maxilla is composed of two irregular bones, which form the bulk of the upper jaw and support the upper teeth. This part of the jaw structure is stationary.

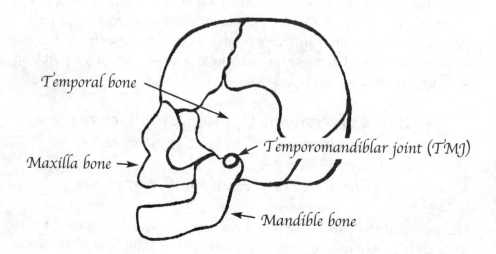

Temporal bone

Temporomandiblar joint (TMJ)

Maxilla bone →

← Mandible bone

The strongest bone in the head is the mandible – the lower jawbone – which is located below the maxilla. This bone supports the bottom teeth. The mandible is hinged to a temporal bone on either side of the skull. This is called the temporomandiblar joint (TMJ). The joint is designed so the lower jaw (mandible) can move from side to side, laterally, as well as up and down, making it a diarthroidal (freely movable) joint.

A good chewing surface is called an occlusion. Occlusion is the meeting of the top and bottom teeth in harmony, the bite or alignment of teeth. Most children have good occlusion with their primary teeth. But when their permanent teeth come in, there is a tendency for crowding and misalignment because the new teeth are larger. The early loss of a primary tooth can cause poor occlusion, or malocclusion, because it acts as a guide for the permanent tooth.

Malocclusion is an abnormal meeting of the teeth or misalignment of the teeth. It can result from several situations – a tooth may erupt in the wrong position, a tooth may be missing, or the child may have two rows of teeth. Some conditions associated with malocclusion include difficulty in chewing, digestion problems, poor speech development, poor aesthetics, pain to the TMJ, damage to the supporting structures and periodontal disease.

The primary teeth are essential to the development of proper speech. The tongue uses the lingual (inside) surface of the upper front teeth for the correct production of many sounds and words. If these teeth are lost through poor dental hygiene or a trauma, a child may have problems pronouncing certain sounds and words.

How Correctional Appliances Effect the Cranium and Facial Structures

◆ The Cranium & How it Works ◆

The relationship between teeth and the cranial bones is significant. The teeth are the fulcrum, or support system of the skull where the whole cranial vault rests and bears weight. It is hinged by the temporomandibular joint. The teeth serve as a support for the cranial structures and have a big influence on the entire body's balance. To fully appreciate what is involved in the process of orthodontic treatment, it helps to understand how the cranium works. The following information simplifies a complex and intricate subject.

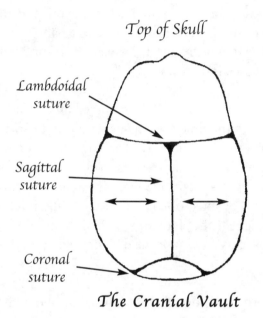

Top of Skull

Lambdoidal
suture

Sagittal
suture

Coronal
suture

The Cranial Vault

The Cranial Rhythm

As the child breathes in and out the cranial bones expand and contract with a free-flowing movement. If there is a restriction in this movement the flow is interrupted, thus interfering with the cranio sacral rhythm of the body.

All of the bones and sutures in the cranium have a free-flowing rhythm. The cranium is the skull, the bony part that encloses the brain. The skull is composed of cranial bones that form a vault for the brain. The bones of the skull move in a synchronistic pattern with the bones of the pelvis to pump cerebrospinal fluid in the spinal column to the brain. This process coordinates neurotransmitters and maintains normal body function. The rhythm of the craniosacral flow is generated by the cyclic production and reabsorption of the cerebrospinal fluid.

If anything interferes with this delicate balance of fluid, the body can malfunction on different levels. If there is a trauma to the head and a restriction occurs, the flow of fluid to the brain becomes inhibited and the sutures get locked-up and stay that way until they are released through some form of manual manipulation.[1]

✦ Misshapen Head or Positional Plagiocephaly ✦

During birth, as the baby travels through the birth canal, the cranium is compressed. It is actually constructed so it will fold over itself. As the infant comes through the birth canal, all the cranial sutures overlap as the head is squashed together. This birthing passage often causes a baby's head to appear pointy or elongated. After birth, the head usually resumes its natural expansion, but in some cases it does not.

Rowan Richards, D.C., a specialist working with developmentally disabled children, believes that a majority of the time the expansion doesn't happen and states, "In examining newborns I would say that 10 percent of the babies are fine after birth, whereas the rest have some form of restriction requiring a few minor adjustments to support the head in expanding back to normal." Cranial distortions occur most often as a result of the infant's position in utero; pressing against the mother's pelvis bone during delivery; being in a cramped space as a twin; or the delivery being too fast or slow.

If the cranial vault doesn't return to a normal, full expansion, the dental arch and teething process can be affected. These children usually develop very narrow, high dental arches. Evidence of this is found where the center of the arch is pointed down and indented. You can actually feel a lump in the middle of the roof of the mouth. This is called a toruspalatinas and is considered normal medically speaking, but according to Richards, not normal in terms of cranial biomechanics.[2]

Another suspected reason for infants' misshapen heads surfaced in 1992, when, in an effort to decrease the cases of sudden infant death syndrome (SIDS) in the United States, the American Academy of Pediatrics (AAP) implemented a "back to sleep" campaign, encouraging parents to place the child on his back to sleep. As a consequence of so many babies being placed on their backs to sleep in the past decade, there has been a high incidence of cranial distortions diagnosed as positional plagiocephaly. Positional plagiocephaly usually happens within the first few weeks after birth as a result of the child being placed on his back for long periods of time, from the head repeatedly resting against a flat surface or from weak neck muscles. Recognizable features of this condition are a flattening of one side or the back of the head, one cheek or ear being noticeably fuller or higher than the other, or the nose being pushed to one side. The face and head are not symmetrical.

Weak neck muscles, or torticollis, occurs when the neck muscles are too tight, have inadequate tone or are shorter on one side or the other, causing the head to remain tilted. Positional plagiocephaly should not be confused with craniosynostosis, which occurs when there is a premature fusion of the seams or sutures between the bony plates in the skull. Proper diagnosis is essential because the routine course of treatment for craniosynostosis is usually surgery. If there is a mistake in the diagnoses and surgery is performed unnecessarily, the consequences are irreversible. In February 1996, an article in the *Wall Street Journal* alerted the public to this growing epidemic of unnecessary cranial surgeries taking place in infants today.[3]

The first recommendation of treatment for positional plagiocephaly is a non-invasive method of repositioning: alternating both your child's direction in the crib and his head position during sleep, and moving objects he likes to look at to different focal locations. During waking hours be sure to put the infant on his tummy periodically when you are interacting with him. If the cause of cranial distortion is due to torticollis, a physical therapist can usually design a home exercise program teaching appropriate neck muscle stretching techniques to help resolve the problem.

Sometimes the cosmetic appearance becomes an issue for parents, prompting them to choose a more invasive approach of remolding the child's head with the use of a helmet. The child wears the helmet for 23 hours a day. This method of treatment, unfortunately, does not address or resolve the actual physical problems, only the cosmetic. If your child is displaying any of these symptoms, my suggestion is to investigate cranial and chiropractic solutions before using invasive techniques.

An infant who has trouble nursing (i.e., difficulty sucking or latching on), is irritable, wants to nurse all the time, or has problems sleeping may have some type of cranial restriction. As the child gets older, these restrictions may contribute to other problems such as developmental delays.[4]

• Cranial Therapy •

Cranial adjustments are the manual manipulation of any restriction of motion in the body's craniosacral rhythm. The adjustment releases the restriction and opens up the sphenoid wings, allowing the whole structure to develop normally. The best window of opportunity to start this work is before the age of 4 years, especially for those with serious cranial problems or a lot of neurological defects. A child's bone structure is more pliable before this age and the problem is easier to correct. The body is more receptive to accepting an adjustment, rather than rejecting it. It is never too late however, to have cranial therapy – even adults can benefit.

This type of adjustment is not invasive and is accomplished with fingertip or thumb pressure. The amount of pressure used, even on newborns, is very gentle. There are several different forms of treatment performed by chiropractors and craniosacral therapists – directional non-force technique, craniosacral therapy, network spinal analysis, etc. It is important to look for a health care practitioner who treats the whole body and has experience in working with infants and children.

• Theories on Crooked Teeth •

In the field of orthodontics, there are different views as to the cause of teeth irregularities in children. Most traditional orthodontists feel that the size of the teeth and dimensions of the jaw are largely predetermined by genetics. Some orthodontists however, who have a more holistic view believe that diet and environment, plus genetics are the ingredients for determining the outcome.

• Sleep & Facial Structure •

Hal Huggins, D.D.S., author of *Why Raise Ugly Kids*, has some intriguing concepts about sleep and facial structure. Huggins interviewed five doctors for his book in an attempt to further confirm his theory of a relationship between sleeping posture and skeletal abnormalities. He concluded that if pressure is applied to a child's bones, the bones will move. Huggins combines the research of Weston Price, D.D.S., and Harvey Stallard, D.D.S., with his own studies and observations in a concise and educational light.

Stallard earned doctorates in education, agriculture, dentistry and orthodontics. He joined a group of pediatricians and staff members of the San Diego City and County Health Department in the 1920s to study changes and development of children's facial structures. The staggering number of 6,772 children of various racial backgrounds were observed over an eight-year period, ranging in age from birth to 17 years old. At the end of the study the doctors said, "Most babies at birth have a few faults in their (facial/cranial) forms, but after 12 months, many have serious faults." Stallard's main interests were in the changes that occurred in the first two years of life. He found that 98 percent had normal facial development at birth and the other 2 percent had "congenital malformations."[5]

It was observed that in the first two years facial structure malformation jumped from 2 to 50 percent, which was a large increase in a short amount of time. There was only an 18 percent increase over the next 15 years, showing how soft and malleable the bones are in an infant and young child.[6]

Stallard's observations showed that improper facial development was associated with specific abnormal pressures during sleep in more than 7,000 cases. Children grow when they are sleeping and are most vulnerable during this time. He witnessed firsthand that many of the orthodontic problems were one sided in direct correlation to specific sleep positions. The cause was a result of different pressures applied to the head while sleeping. Stallard considered hands, fingers, knuckles, arms and pillows to be the orthodontic appliances that work against you. For instance, if there is pressure on the side of the skull from a pillow, or hand pushing on the orbit of the eye socket, the development of its full roundedness can be jeopardized. An eye that is not fully rounded is called astigmatism. These pressures cause structural changes in the skull, such as narrow faces, depressed cheekbones, small chins and crowded teeth.[7]

Stallard's theories of posture and sleep positions are worth further investigation. He felt that a stomach-sleeper would tend to be more stooped over, have shoulder blades that stick out like wings, and a head that falls forward with a narrow face. When you sleep on your stomach, you turn your head to one side or the other, putting pressure on one side of the facial structures causing a long narrowing effect. This also pushes up the palate causing a high, narrow palatal vault.

Stomach-sleepers often develop both orthodontic and orthopedic problems. Stallard states, "Orthodontic problems are those limited to tooth positions. Orthopedic problems are those limited to bones. Unfortunately, the bones being affected contain teeth – therefore, we have an overlapping orthodontic-orthopedic problem." He felt someone who sleeps on his stomach has a much higher incidence of distortion to the facial bones that interfere with growth patterns. Also, babies are belly breathers and if you place them to sleep on their stomachs, their breathing isn't as fluid as it should be.[8]

The pillow stacker forces the head out of its midline position. This is evident from the tilt of the head when they face someone standing by the bed. The positioning of the hand against the face can cause teeth to be pushed back. In some cases this can result in one tooth being behind the rest of the teeth. If the hand is pushing on the lower teeth in a repetitive pattern night after night, it can stunt the growth of the lower jaw or again push the teeth backward. Stallard believed that sleeping on the stomach "prevents the genetic potential from fulfilling its role."

Stallard found that side sleepers encouraged the spine to develop with one long curve in it. One shoulder blade sticks out, and the hands are usually placed against the face putting pressure on the developing face. He thought this pressure on the nose would influence the molars and back teeth, and could lead to nasal septum deviation.

Back-sleepers stand tall and proud with excellent posture, and usually have good teeth developing equally on both sides. Those who sleep on their backs also have straight spines. Stallard believed that the full effect of a genetic potential could only be achieved by sleeping on the back. "Mash those faces and you have crooked teeth, crooked noses, undeveloped cheek bones, small lower jaws, receding chins – even visual problems." He was convinced that certain sleeping positions were responsible for robbing the mouth of adequate room for the third molars or wisdom teeth.[9]

◆ *The Effects of Nutrition On* ◆ *Facial Development*

Weston Price, D.D.S., author of *Nutrition and Physical Degeneration*, was a pioneer in linking diet and nutrition to chronic and degenerative diseases in the body. He observed that his younger patients had increasingly deformed dental arches, crooked teeth and cavities. In his studies, he found that women with poor diets of modern foods (sugar, white flour, convenience foods) produced children with long narrow faces, crowded teeth and pinched noses. Equally as damaging were children raised on the same diet, which created similar facial irregularities.

Price's research showed that dental arches failed to attain their full genetic development when certain fats were missing from the diet, which he felt was because the intestinal tract is a fat-soluble membrane and requires the presence of fat to properly absorb its nutrients (minerals). So when the body is lacking in good fat, the end result will be a nutritional deficiency, affecting the bones and teeth. Price and Stallard both recognized a biochemical nutritional cause behind improper development.[10]

In his book, Price discusses the use of butter concentrate to increase mineral absorption. He found that as butter was increased in the diet, blood levels of calcium and inorganic phosphorous improved, consequently improving facial structures. His research showed that there was an unknown fat substance in butter associated with a resistance to decay and the stimulation of bone growth. This fatty substance had some similar characteristics as vitamins A and D, both fat-soluble vitamins. If the diet was low in this nutrient, Price observed that the lateral incisors (number two from the midline) were set in toward the palate and the cuspids were more outward to the lip.[11]

Dentist Hal Huggins, D.D.S., corroborated Price's findings within his own practice. He found that he could tell whether a child had been raised on margarine or butter. Huggins states, "If the kid was raised on butter, his facial form and tooth position were markedly better than those raised on margarine, regardless of sleeping habits."

In addition to affecting the development of the jaw and teeth it was noted that proper levels of fat in the diet also helped the body to achieve orthodontic correction quicker in realigning teeth. Price states, "In the movement of teeth consideration of mineral metabolism should be prime."

◆ *Posture & Facial Development* ◆

Orthodontist David Berrios, D.D.S., believes that structural changes occur as a result of upper body posture, breathing technique and swallowing patterns. He states, "In my practice, I would say 95 percent of my patients have malocclusion as a result of their posture. If children are all hunched over in the shoulder and neck area with their mouths hanging open, teeth and facial structures will suffer."

The optimal growth pattern for correct facial posture occurs when the mouth is closed and breathing takes place through the nose. The lips gently meet and the tongue rests on the soft palate located in the roof of the mouth away from the teeth. The tongue placement and swallowing patterns act as a guide for the teeth and jaw development. This positioning allows the teeth to slide into the correct spot as they erupt, and the muscles in the face to be properly trained.

If the child is a mouth breather, the mouth will hang open, influencing all aspects of the facial structure: the shape of the face, the nose, throat, spacing for the teeth, even the tooth's susceptibility to decay, due to a decrease of saliva production, which protects the teeth.

When teeth erupt they continue growing until they meet a resistance – other teeth. If the mouth is open most of the time teeth grow beyond their means, causing an improper bite alignment. Children who spend a majority of the time breathing through the mouth will develop long faces by encouraging the jaw to grow downward, narrowing the dental arch and crowding teeth. If the child maintains a correct facial posture, the jaw will grow forward and expand out, supporting a good-looking face, jaw line and smile.

Inadvertent habits, like jaw leaning, thumb or finger sucking, etc., also encourage abnormal and unattractive growth patterns. Most research has found that once an abnormal pattern establishes itself, it will continue unless there is some form of intervention.

◆ Correcting the Problem ◆
Small Mouths & Crooked Teeth

The process of realigning teeth with a corrective device works by gentle pressure. The socket or hole the tooth is housed in is a living bone and can be changed with pressure, leaving the bone or tooth unharmed.

There are different techniques used to straighten teeth. The two most common practices are traditional orthodontics and dental orthopedics. Orthodontic means to straighten teeth, and dental orthopedics refers to moving the jaw. There is, however, another technique that is not as well known called orthotropics, which is the science of guiding the growth of the facial structures. Orthodontists who are qualified to practice this form of "growth guidance" have several additional years of this specific training.

◆ Orthodontics ◆

In the field of orthodontics or teeth straightening, there are three classes in the distinction of malocclusion:

Class I –   crowded teeth, normal jaws
Class II –   buckteeth; weak chin indicating receding jaw
Class III –   bulldog jaw, protrusive jaws; thrust forward;
              lower teeth in front of upper

There are two phases to orthodontic work. The first phase is called preventative or interceptive orthodontics and involves the introduction of doctor to patient and the assessment orientation. This can take place anytime between 6 and 9 years of age. Treatment options can be explored, discussed and, in certain instances, even implemented at this time to prepare the child's mouth for future work.

If the mouth is too small and there is crowding, the first course of action in traditional orthodontics is the use of a rapid palatable expander. (Alternatives for this treatment will be introduced in following sections.) The expander is cemented in the roof of the mouth where it is used to widen the palate to create more space for the teeth. There is a screw located in its center, which is turned by a key once or twice a day to expand the walls of the jaw outward.

The time needed to accomplish this expansion process varies depending on the child. Usually the course of treatment takes between three and five months, but in certain instances, can take over a year. Once this phase is completed, a retainer may be used to maintain the change until the age of 12 when the bones become more fixed and solid, or until the second phase of treatment begins, if needed, which involves the placement of braces.

Another consideration during the early years is if the child loses a tooth prematurely, a space maintainer or lingual arch can be worn to prevent other teeth from drifting into the empty space.

The second phase of the work usually begins between 10 and 12 years depending on where the child is in the teething process and the extent of work that needs to be done. Braces and (the sometimes needed) headgear are the traditional correctional appliances used during this phase.

◆ *Braces* ◆

Braces are a non-removable orthodontic appliance used to correct misaligned teeth or malocclusion. They are made up of bands, brackets and wires. The bands are the foundation, and are individually placed around key teeth involved in the realigning process. For some kids, this means all teeth. Sometimes, wedge-shaped spacers are used to help make room for the bands if the teeth are too close together.

Brackets are bonded to the teeth, and depending on the orthodontist or aesthetics, the hardware can be used on either the outside or inside of the tooth (most commonly on the outer surface). One or more arch wires are then passed through the brackets and extended to the bands, tying the teeth together. The tightening of the wires produces movement of the teeth for corrections. There are several options regarding bracket material – the traditional silver wire, clear, glow in the dark, fad colors or tooth-colored plastic.

One drawback of using braces is that when teeth are bound together the craniosacral rhythm usually becomes restricted. Some of the symptoms associated with these restrictions occur after an adjustment of the braces and include tenderness of jaw, teeth, ear areas, headache, inability to concentrate, etc.

Another problem is that the two metals used in the composition of braces contain nickel and chromium. Both are known to have cancer-causing properties. According to Frank J. Jerome, D.D.S., author of *Tooth Truth*, some children may be hypersensitive to nickel and display symptoms such as depression, dropping grades, personality changes and in rare cases, urinary tract problems due to a growth of nickel-dependent bacteria.[12]

If unusual or persistent symptoms occur, a compatibility test can be taken (for a fee) that will tell if your child is allergic or sensitive to the metals. For more details on the test, call the Huggins Diagnostic Center at 800-331-2303.

Children who wear braces should avoid sticky foods like gum, taffy and caramel and hard crunchy foods like corn chips, popcorn and nuts. Other hard foods like fruits, vegetables and bread crusts can be cut into bite-size pieces.

Self-help:
The most common homeopathic remedies to be considered after a child's

braces have been tightened are: *Arnica, Hypericum, Chamomilla* or *Ferrum phosphoricum.*

Most children and teenagers also benefit from a chiropractic or cranial adjustment following a visit to the orthodontist.

◆ *Headgear* ◆

A headgear appliance is used if the front teeth need to be pulled back because of an overbite, and is most often worn at night. From a holistic viewpoint, this type of restriction to the facial structure interferes with the body's natural growth process and in addition to being uncomfortable, can create a flat face.

◆ *Orthotropics* ◆

There are many different types of special appliances and systems for the treatment of abnormal facial and dental growth patterns in children. The following alternative techniques are similar in their philosophy of supporting a more gentle process for proper facial development and teeth alignment.

In 1958, orthodontist John Mew, D.D.S., introduced the "Tropic Premise" which suggested that irregular teeth were not necessarily hereditary, but rather the result of poor oral posture. He believed that oral habits were responsible for guiding the jaw and teeth into proper occlusion and that the direction of facial growth has a strong influence on the end result.

The preferred direction of growth is horizontal. Mew thought that traditional braces support vertical growth and only treat the symptoms of malocclusion rather than the cause, producing flat faces. After years of frustration with the old methods, he developed orthotropics or "growth guidance" and the Biobloc system of treatment.

The philosophy behind orthotropics is to encourage growth guidance, to support the mouth in developing to its full potential, thus making enough room for all of the permanent teeth. When this is accomplished, tooth extractions and surgery are typically not necessary.

If a child develops poor oral posture and/or habits that interfere with the natural growth process, resulting in tooth misalignment, proper intervention is critical. The Biobloc system is a holistic approach to the problem. The goal of the system is to correct the environmental problems by using an appliance to strengthen jaw muscles and train the child to keep his mouth closed. It encourages a forward or horizontal growth of the face instead of a downward or vertical growth.

The Biobloc is a device that fits in the palate and, like the palatable expander, has a screw in the center, which is rotated by a key daily. But instead of just pushing outward like its traditional counterpart, it expands in all directions and can be removed. In addition to promoting proper oral posture the appliance lifts and intrudes permanent teeth, alleviating big, gummy smiles.

There are four stages to the Biobloc system and treatment can begin shortly after all the primary teeth have erupted, as early as 6 years old. Not every child requires all four stages; it depends on the amount of correction needed. One of the drawbacks to the Biobloc is that its success depends on the child's participation and commitment. Depending on the age at which a child starts the process, it can sometimes take longer than the traditional route. But if you start when the child is young and their bones are still pliable and soft, the goal can be achieved quicker.

Complements to the Biobloc system are the shared benefits of Crozat therapy and myofunctional exercises. Some of the exercises used to retrain poor oral posture include: holding a paper clip gently between the lips while resting the mid-tongue on the roof of the mouth, away from the teeth and practice swallowing; putting a small rubber band on the tongue and holding it against the roof of the mouth while swallowing. The child can practice one of these exercises for a few hours each day to help improve unhealthy tongue habits, breathing techniques and to support proper growth.

See pictures on page 212

◆ Crozat Therapy ◆

Most people have never heard of the Crozat correction technique, developed and perfected by George B. Crozat, D.D.S., more than 70 years ago in New Orleans. The appliance is constructed of a thin wire, usually of precious metal rather than steel (some of the wires do contain a percentage of nickel), custom fit to the child's mouth. It generally fits on the inside of the teeth, on the roof of the mouth, or under the tongue. The Crozat appliance, similar to the Biobloc system, encourages and guides the growth of the bony structure that supports the teeth. For most of the treatment, there are no visible signs that the child is wearing an appliance. Depending on the situation, sometimes a wire might have to be run along the outside of the teeth as well.

Mark Harmon, D.D.S., states, "Malocclusions usually go hand-in-hand with mouths and faces that are too small. Therefore, a corrective force applied from the inside is the most efficient way to expand outward in all directions. This is also done without requiring teeth to be tied to neighboring teeth as used in conventional orthodontic treatment, restricting desirable free movement of the teeth."[13]

It is rare that a tooth would have to be extracted with the guidance of Crozat therapy, as the object is to make room for all the teeth. The appliance actually helps the bones and muscles of the face and jaw to grow naturally and develop fully.

The Crozat wire is a removable appliance, which requires an adjustment by the dentist or orthodontist approximately every two to four weeks to widen, rotate and position the teeth. It applies mild pressure to the appropriate teeth in the right place, at the right time.[14]

See pictures on page 213

• *Advanced Lightwire Functional or ALF* •

Another alternative device for correcting orthodontic/orthopedic problems is the Advanced Lightwire Functional or the ALF. Darick Nordstrom, D.D.S., developed the concept and design of the ALF in 1982, with the influence of Crozat and Kernott (not discussed in this book) as its springboards. He wanted to create an appliance that would support the osteopathic principles of keeping the premaxilla and facial bones free flowing and unrestricted, which allowed him to use the most natural, gentle force possible during orthodontic correction. The ALF has a lighter, springier wire with half or one-third the thickness of other conventional wires. The wire's individualized design helps realign the underlying cranial distortions responsible for particular orthodontic/orthopedic problems. The loops on the appliance that make it springy also train the tongue, which induces the patient to swallow properly, resolving tongue-thrusting issues more rapidly. It is considered a removable fixed appliance that remains stationary in the child's mouth for treatment, but is sometimes removed during office evaluation and adjustment. The appliance is readjusted at each visit in conjunction with cranial manipulation to facilitate healthy movement of the skull bones. This dual action assists in reducing the relapse patterns of the teeth to old, crooked positions (and cranial distortions) and supports a more normal neurological and spinal function. According to Murdock Laboratories, the manufacturer, it is a versatile appliance that can be used in virtually any configuration.

The only change in eating habits for both the Crozat and the ALF systems are no chewing gum or sticky candy and to use caution when biting into hard foods, such as French bread crusts. Check with your dentist for other restrictions that might need to be considered.

The actual costs vary with each child, as well as the amount of time needed to complete the correction process, depending on the extent of the problem. For more information on the ALF you can contact Nordstrom at darick@nordstromd.com.

See pictures on page 214

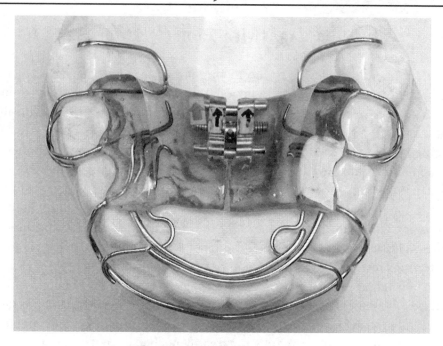

Biobloc – first stage, sample

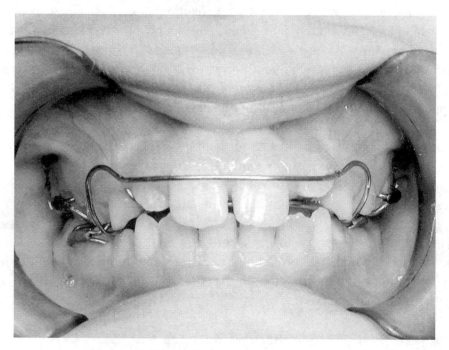

Biobloc – first stage, front view

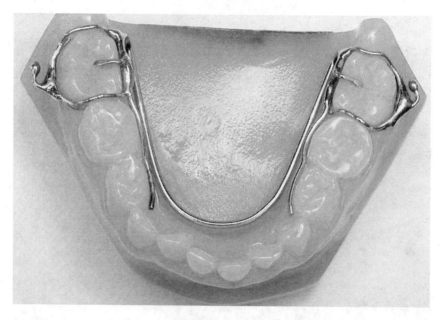

Crozat sample

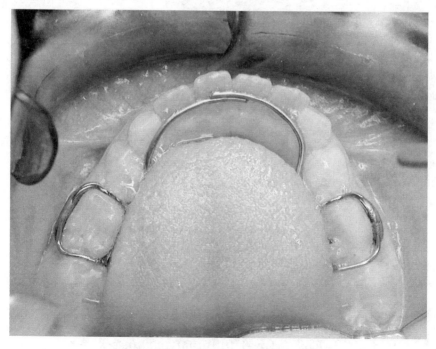

Crozat – bottom appliance

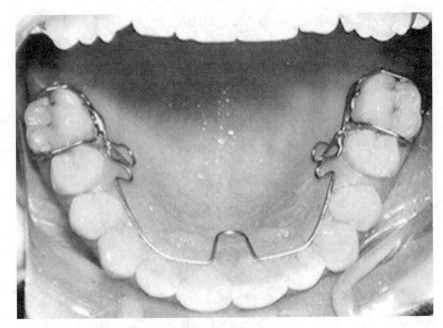

Advanced Lightwire Functional or ALF - Upper

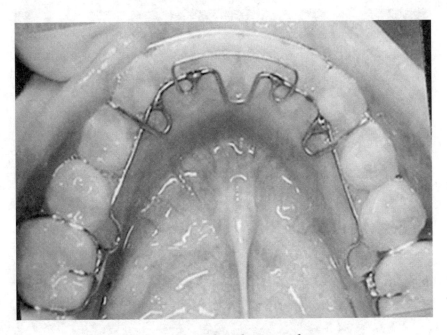

ALF - Lower finishing appliance

♦ Hygiene: Correctional Appliances ♦

Whichever form of corrective appliance you choose for your child, hygiene is of the utmost importance. Food, germs and plaque create a toxic environment in the mouth contributing to cavities and gum disease. With stationary appliances such as braces, flossing is not possible; however, the ALF is so small and non-intrusive that you actually can floss easily, and in most cases with the crozat appliance as well. All three of these appliances benefit from water irrigation, but it is essential with braces. Always check with the dentist, orthodontist or hygienist regarding proper use of a water irrigation instrument while wearing a correctional appliance. Ask for directional guidance and appropriate speed settings to use for optimal results. *(See chapter on "Keeping Teeth Clean.")*

Conclusion

If the child needs a correctional appliance, it is good practice to schedule chiropractic and or cranial adjustments in conjunction with the orthodontic work. Rowan Richards, D.C., feels the adjustments encourage the teeth to move quicker, achieving a faster correction, as well as minimizing or alleviating physical symptoms such as, headaches, lack of concentration, sore throat, etc.

If your child experiences emotional and/or physical symptoms after the introduction of some form of dental work or correctional appliance, investigate the possibilities – there could be a sensitivity to the materials being used, or perhaps the rhythmic plates in the cranium have become restricted (locked up) or damaged as a result of the work. If a restriction does occur, the child may need a chiropractic or cranial adjustment to rectify the problem.

A sensitive child may experience problems with concentration (displaying similar behavior to that of attention deficit disorder, or ADD), signs of hyperactivity, or he may become more susceptible to illness within days following an adjustment to a correctional appliance (i.e., a cold, headache, earache, stomach distress, etc.). Become an observant parent so you can recognize a problem early and remedy it accordingly.

"The tooth fairy has a nice pretty gown, feathery wings, and a bow on top of her head and comes in through the window. She lives in a pretty forest called the Rainbow Forest. Her house is made out of flowers and teeth. She puts a flower between each tooth. Since she needs the teeth, she thinks it is fair to leave something like a present or money. The bigger the teeth the more cool stuff she leaves. Her walkway is made from beautiful stones and the furniture from diamonds. She is adding on to her house so she really needs the teeth to make more room in case visitors come over. She wants us to have grown up teeth."

Kailia - 7 years old: lots of missing teeth

"I lost my first tooth at school and my teacher put it in a pouch for me to take home. I put my tooth in a little bitty fairy box that opens by the side of my bed. The next morning the tooth fairy brought me some bulbs wrapped up in paper – you know they grow into flowers. But I didn't know what they would look like so my mommy helped me plant them. I waited a long time, but when they grew, they turned into giant pink Dahlia flowers and every year they bloom again. She also brought me roses for another tooth – that tooth fairy has a thing about garden flowers. There are lots of different tooth fairies – there is the garden one, the stone one, the feather one, and the crystal one. I don't understand why the tooth fairy brings so many different kinds of things. Sometimes, I want a different fairy than the one that comes, but usually I do like what she brings."

Selina - 8 years old

Chapter Ten

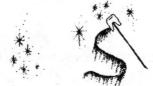

Personal Stories & Case Studies

◆ Examining the Relationship Between ◆ Teething, Illness & Behavior

The following stories and observations are meant to offer greater insight into the correlation between the teething process and different physical and emotional symptoms or behaviors.

The first section describes some of the teething-related symptoms my daughter Danielle has experienced over the years. It was through my observations of these symptoms in relation to her teeth that I decided to write this book. She is 18 years old now, still teething (wisdom teeth) and continues to display many different symptoms – physical, emotional and behavioral. Her "Dr. Jekyll and Ms. Hyde" behavior has accompanied the eruption or loss of almost every tooth throughout her life. The second section is a compilation of parents' personal stories I have chronicled describing their children's physical and emotional behaviors during the teething process.

◆ Danielle 's Personal Story ◆

Danielle had trouble teething with every tooth in her mouth. The ones that created the most problems were the 2-, 6- and 12-year molars. When her molars were coming in the symptoms were always more intense, including ear infections, drooling, croup, coughs, sinus, teeth grinding and sleeplessness.

By the age of 2 months, Danielle was already experiencing gas, drooling and irritability. Her first tooth, however, wasn't visible until 5 months. The 6-year molars started coming in at 4 1/2 years, the 12-year molars at 10 years and her wisdom teeth at the age of 15 1/2. In observing my clients and daughter's friends over the years, I have found that 60 to 70 percent of the girls get their teeth earlier than the boys.

◆ Ear Infections ◆

It took me three years to realize that Danielle's ear infections were not bacterial, but rather related to food allergies and teething. She was 5 months old when she was diagnosed with her first ear infection and given antibiotics. That is also when her first tooth erupted. This was the beginning of what would become years of chronic health problems – croup, ear infections, enlarged tonsils, a suppressed immune system, nightmares, environmental, chemical and food sensitivities, with repeated courses of antibiotics and other drugs. As I learned more about the immune system, it became clear that the repeated use of antibiotics was actually compromising her health during the teething process. I knew then it was time to find a new way of addressing her physical symptoms.

Danielle took her last round of antibiotics just before her third birthday and I spent the next year rebuilding her damaged immune system. She remained healthy for the a few years until her 6-year molars started to come in and she developed another ear infection. Instead of reverting back to antibiotics we used homeopathic remedies, herbal eardrops and vitamin supplements. From that point on, she never needed another antibiotic despite the continuance of many of the symptoms covered in these pages.

♦ *Drooling, Coughs, Croup, Sinus,* ♦ *Sleeplessness, & Teeth grinding*

Danielle started drooling excessively at around 4 months and didn't stop until her 2-year molars were completely in. In our mothers group, she was known as the "drool queen." When her 6-year molars started erupting the drooling reoccurred. As she got older, instead of the saliva dribbling down her chin, it would run down the back of her throat and create a cough. Her teething coughs would express in different ways – dry, wet, sporadic, persistent, with her sinuses alternating between stuffy and running like a faucet, lasting anywhere from one day to a month.

Most recently, as her second wisdom tooth started poking through the gum, she experienced a dry persistent cough and a stuffy nose for about three weeks, and her moods fluctuated between happy or sweet and totally irrational and out of control.

Danielle has gotten croup with the eruption of almost every tooth, including her 12-year molars and wisdom teeth. Most children grow out of the croup stage once they have all their primary teeth, but Danielle fell into a different category – the small percentage of kids that continue to get croup through their teenage years.

Despite what experts say, Danielle's sleep patterns have always been affected by her teething. Between 18 and 24 months she would wake up inconsolable in the middle of the night. As she grew, the behavior continued on and off for months with the eruption of each molar. Even now as her wisdom teeth are coming in, she is still quite wakeful for weeks at a time. Once each set of molars were in, her sleep patterns would return to normal. Danielle can almost always be made more comfortable with the appropriate homeopathic remedy.

Teeth grinding or bruxism is another common occurrence for a teething child. Danielle started grinding her teeth as soon as she had two on the top and two on the bottom. Her grinding became so severe when her 6-year molars were erupting that the noise would keep me up at night.

✦ Stomachaches ✦

When Danielle was 5 years old, I learned firsthand how intricate the relationship really is between teeth and the rest of the body. One day when I picked her up from school, she complained of a stomachache. The subject was dropped until just before bed when she mentioned it again, but was able to fall asleep. Around midnight I woke up to her piercing cry, "My tummy hurts," at which point I called her pediatrician immediately.

There were no other symptoms, no fever, gas, vomiting or sweating. The pain was located directly around her navel. Eventually, she was able to fall back to sleep and was fine the next morning. As a precaution I took her to the pediatrician, who ordered several blood tests. By mid afternoon the pain returned. This time I called our homeopathic doctor and explained the situation. He saw us immediately and sent us home with three different remedies. After the first remedy she seemed much better – she ate dinner, was happy, playful and once again everything seemed normal.

She fell asleep for a few hours before the pain returned, which kept us up most of the night. The next morning while lying in bed she announced, "It feels like there's a string tied from my tooth to my tummy."

Having had very little sleep, I didn't give much thought to her words. Later that afternoon however, I had a dentist appointment and took her along. Danielle was in the process of losing her first tooth, so I asked the dentist if it was possible for a loose tooth to cause this obscure pain. The dentist assured me there was no connection between the two.

All of the tests ordered by her pediatrician came back normal. Four days of discomfort and the doctors were still baffled. Even though Danielle's bowel movements were normal, her pediatrician suggested we seek the advice of a gastrointestinal specialist to rule out any type of intestinal blockage. The diagnosis was normal, the cure, a prescription for an anti-spasmodic medication. Needless to say, I was very frustrated by this point.

On the way home, Danielle again mentioned that she felt like there was a connection between her tooth and her tummy. This time I listened to her and decided to treat the pain as though it were related to the tooth. When we got home, I made a mouthwash out of a liquid tincture for teeth related problems and had her rinse with the solution. Within five minutes she was asleep and rested comfortably for three hours. When she woke up, I then tried a homeopathic remedy for nerve pain and she slept through the rest of the night for the first time in five days. When the pain returned a few days later, I repeated the remedy. After that she remained pain free until she started losing her second tooth. Fortunately, by that time we knew what to do.

When I shared the story with a friend, Lynne Walker, a pharmacist, acupuncturist and homeopath, she explained that in Chinese medicine there are meridians, or invisible channels, which travel through and around the entire body. They are the carriers or circulators of life force energy, or chi. Meridians are believed to run parallel to each other and travel along nerve pathways throughout the human body. Walker explained that there was definitely a connection via these meridians between the tooth and Danielle's stomach pain.

In 15 years I have met a handful of other children who experienced the same pain with the loss of their first tooth. Never, however, ignore a child complaining of stomach pain. As you can see from my family's personal story, we thoroughly examined all possibilities to rule out a more serious health problem. If a child is experiencing pain of any kind, always seek the advice of a medical doctor immediately.

Attention Deficit Hyperactive Disorder (ADHD) & Attention Deficit Disorder (ADD)

When Danielle was in middle school, I was shocked to find that 98 percent of her male classmates had been diagnosed with ADHD or ADD and were on one of many prescription drugs (i.e. Ritalin, Dexedrine, Cylert, etc.). The reality of this mass medication program was disturbing.

If Danielle had actually undergone analysis, my suspicion is that she too would have been diagnosed with ADHD. She was notorious for displaying many of the symptoms listed in the *Diagnostic & Statistical Manual of*

Mental Disorders or DSM-IV. From the time she was born, she was wired energetically and in constant motion. Teachers' comments always expressed the same: "Talks too much, missing assignments and unable to concentrate."

Discovering the source behind her behavior became an enlightening journey for me. I found there were three major components: The influence of the teething process; a problem with food allergies (i.e. sugar, dairy, dyes, preservatives, etc.) or environmental sensitivities (either nature's influence or chemical based); and parasites and/or an excess of yeast in the intestinal tract. *(See chapter on "Teething Related Symptoms.")*

◆ Crozat Therapy ◆

When Danielle was 9, our dentist presented us with two options for correcting crooked teeth – the traditional method of braces or a more holistic approach, with the Crozat wire. Because of Danielle's sensitive nature, we decided to go with the least intrusive appliance – the Crozat method.

With my daughter's treatment, the appliance was stationary except for the few times she dislodged it with her tongue by accident. When that happened the dentist needed to inspect it to make sure it wasn't damaged and reposition it securely in her mouth. Danielle wore her Crozat appliance for approximately 11 months and the cost was comparable to other orthodontic appliances, such as braces. The most effective hygiene tool while wearing the Crozat (in addition to brushing) was the use of a water irrigation system.

◆ Brushing Teeth ◆

Getting a child to brush their teeth at any age can be a real challenge. To my preteen, a 10 second movement of the brush was considered good brushing. Obviously, this was not good hygiene practice and eventually we came up with a formula that worked for all of us – a radio in the bathroom with the agreement to brush for an entire song.

By the age of 16, Danielle had realized how important her teeth were and started spending more time devoted to her oral hygiene. When asked why, she replied, "My smile is important to me." She now advises younger children to have fun with brushing and rinsing. "If kids don't take care of their teeth when they are young, they will end up with no teeth, like many grandparents."

◆ Gum Chewing ◆

Danielle had a perfectly clean dental record until she was 8 years old, at which point she suddenly developed five gum-line cavities from one dental visit to the next. The only thing different was she had discovered chewing gum of the sugar variety. The dentist said, "The sudden arrival of multiple cavities is common among sugar-laced gum chewers."

◆ Parents' Personal Stories ◆

Kaeli (3-5 years)

Kaeli never had colds or symptoms of sickness as a baby except when she was teething. She would have one or two bouts of diarrhea and experience a clear, runny nose when a tooth was erupting. We didn't realize the pattern until a few teeth had come through. She was also bratty, stubborn, difficult and whiny.

Kaeli is 5 years old now and her baby teeth are getting ready to fall out. Recently, she started behaving differently. She is very fearful that she will be left alone at night and is having trouble separating from me. It is much harder for her to fall asleep and she is very whiny and fidgety.

Chad (as a baby & older)

When Chad was teething, he wouldn't sleep through the night, which was very difficult on the rest of the family. He drooled a lot from 9 months until he was 3 years old, which periodically caused a ticklish cough. He also had bouts of diarrhea, red gums and a loss of appetite while teething. I don't recall his mood being aggressive like his sisters, but rather sensitive. Now that he is older he still displays this sensitivity, but can also be quite bossy.

Chad is 10 now and to this day the only time he doesn't eat like a horse is when he is teething.

Emma (1-2 years)

She would have a runny nose – like a faucet, for about a week before the eruption of a tooth. Sometimes the stuff coming out of her nose would turn green or yellow in color by the third or fourth day. Her mood was very unhappy, whiny, clingy, etc. She was not able to fall asleep and would be up until 12:30 a.m. just crying, when normally she was a great sleeper. Emma also became quite uncontrollable – she wouldn't stay in her crib and started climbing out during fits of anger, which was very dangerous. She was also a good eater except when she was teething.

When Emma was 2 years old, she constantly had her fingers in her mouth. At times she actually attempted fitting her whole fist in at once. She would put her fingers in her ears, had a runny nose and a sporadic cough (usually at night). These symptoms continued for weeks before one of the molars actually broke through.

Ella (4 years)

The dentist had discovered Ella had four cavities in her molars. They filled one of the cavities during our first visit and suggested we schedule three additional visits to repair the rest of the teeth. The fact that Ella had any cavities at all was a shock because we don't eat sweets or drink sodas. My older son has never had a cavity.

Upon Kathy's recommendation, I started giving Ella homeopathic cell salt remedies and by her next check-up, the dentist felt her teeth had somehow improved and decided not to fill the remaining cavities at that time. After reevaluating her teeth, he requested two additional visits for the year to keep an eye on things. Ella's teeth stabilized and of the original three remaining cavities, only one needed to be filled two years later because of a crack in the tooth. Ella is 6 1/2 years old now.

The physical and emotional symptoms Ella experienced while teething were obvious. When she was around 6, her nose ran constantly, eventually turning green in color and she was very irritable. The first time this happened, the symptoms lasted a few weeks before I called Kathy for advice. I gave Ella a homeopathic remedy for teething and her symptoms cleared up overnight along with her unpleasant disposition. A few days later I realized her first 6-year molar had erupted.

Once all of her molars were in, I thought we were home free, but then she started losing her baby teeth, new permanent ones began coming in and all of the symptoms returned. That's when I realized teething was something my kids would be going through for a long time.

Ilan (3 months-1 year)

Ilan was a very colicky baby who needed a lot of attention. I was concerned about taking a fussy baby on the long plane ride from Israel to the United States. After telling Kathy his symptoms, she felt he might actually be teething already and suggested I try a homeopathic remedy, which worked great for the plane ride and trip.

Then when Ilan was 1 year old, he got sick with the flu. The only thing that would calm him down was nursing. If I put him down, he would just cry continuously. After a few days I tried giving him the homeopathic teething remedy *Chamomilla* and within a half-hour his fever was gone and he fell asleep. When he woke up he was back to normal.

Moe (7 years)

Moe's top front teeth were pulled when he was 2 years old due to bottle-mouth syndrome. He is 7 1/2 years old now and, unfortunately, his adult teeth still haven't grown in. He did, however, lose his front bottom teeth naturally and the new ones have come in just fine. Moe experiences a lot of burping and digestive problems when he is teething and becomes argumentative and bossy.

Maddie (infant-7 years)

When Maddie was a baby and teething, she would repeatedly get earaches, a runny raw nose, diaper rash, fever, croup and bad chest colds where she couldn't breathe at night. She was very sensitive emotionally and would talk back, which was not her usual nature. Once all of her teeth were in, she was very healthy for the next few years. When she started losing her first baby tooth at 7, she suddenly started getting sick again – difficulty breathing, snoring with a stuffy nose and a sore throat. Emotionally she became whiny, began throwing tantrums, was fighting with all of her friends and being very rough – pinching and digging her nails into me. She also started chewing on things like pencils and pens and was having trouble listening. She didn't want to separate from me and complained all the time that it is too hot or that she is tired. Most recently, she had an earache, stuffy nose, sore throat, chapped lips and a rash on the right side of her face. I told Kathy my daughter was acting like she did when she was a baby. That's when Kathy asked if Maddie was getting her molars. So I looked in her mouth and sure enough, she was getting two of them.

Kelsie (7 years)
My daughter is acting very wacky and having trouble listening in school. She can't focus on what people are saying and is having trouble falling asleep. She is angry, yelling a lot and has frequent stomachaches. Her two front teeth are missing on the bottom and the new ones are just starting to erupt.

Casey (10 years)
Last week, Casey kept saying she didn't feel well and missed a field trip. She was very tired and had a sore throat with a fever. Her disposition was cranky and moody. She told me her gums were hurting in the back, so I looked inside her mouth and found that all four of her 12-year molars were coming in at once. Recently, Casey also lost her first molars and her canines are coming in – she is really a mess with this teething.

Andrew (6 years)
When Andrew was a baby, he got croup a lot while he was teething. After all his baby teeth came in he was pretty healthy, but recently he has started getting sick again and there has been a loss of appetite. He has been very frustrated, strong willed and now has a rash all over his face. At night he is fearful and needs me to lay down with him and is experiencing low self-confidence. His last two 6-year molars are getting ready to break through the skin.

Stephen (10 years)

Stephen is teething like crazy. He has a geographic tongue and goes from one nervous habit to another, such as obsessively digging his nails into his cheeks. He is also distracted easily and has trouble concentrating in school. Tantrums are a daily occurrence and he is fearful of the dark. He is getting a lot of new teeth.

Elaina (9 years)

She has several loose teeth and is getting several new ones. She has been sick with a lot of colds lately, is completely stuffed up, has lots of mucus and when she sneezes all this goo comes out. Her self-confidence is down and she doesn't seem to like the changes that accompany growing up. There is a constant fear that I will die, which prevents her from sleeping well at night, and last but not least, daily stomachaches.

Madison (17 months)

She is getting her 2-year molars and has been sick on and off. Her nose is running constantly, alternating between cream and green in color and she has bad breath, a lot of smelly gas, a rash on her tummy, a barking cough, is cranky, does not want to eat and has a goopy eye with yellow discharge.

Lily (7 years)

Lily is getting her eyeteeth and has a sore throat, fever, stuffy nose, croupy cough, bad breath, is wheezing and is very grouchy. These symptoms have been going on for weeks and we have already tried antibiotics – nothing seems to help her.

Carolyn (11 years)

I am very concerned about my daughter. She has so many health and emotional problems: constant stuffy nose, always tired, can't sleep, needs company in the room to fall asleep, has trouble making friends, chews on her fingers, fears intruders, just an overall state of anxiety about everything. Two of her 12-year molars are just coming in.

Shasha (10 years)

She didn't get her first tooth until after her first birthday. When Shasha was seven years old, most of her friends had already lost a few teeth and new ones were coming in. But not hers, as a matter of fact, her permanent teeth started coming in long before she ever had a loose tooth. Consequently, she ended up having two rows of teeth for a long time. She eventually did lose her two top front teeth, but that was because her brother actually knocked them out by accident.

Ireland (6 years)
Every time Ireland has a tooth coming in or falling out her nose either becomes runny or stuffy. I hate to be so graphic, but the goo in her nose turns yellow or green. She gets fevers on and off for no apparent reason, has explosive coughs, mostly at night and can be very grouchy.

Lee (12 years)
His molars are half way in on the bottom and he has a constant sensation of needing to sneeze, but only sneezes once and a while. He has a croupy cough, has waves of nausea, frequent headaches, diarrhea that comes and goes, is lightheaded at times and is having trouble sleeping. Lee feels very stressed and is getting his 12-year molars.

Riley (6 years)
Her top two front teeth are coming in but they haven't broken the skin yet. She has a lot of mucus running down the back of her throat. Her nose is full of green mucus, is raw inside and she also has a cough.

Madison (10 months)
She has already had six ear infections and the doctors just keep giving her antibiotics. Every time she finishes the antibiotic she gets another ear infection. She had six teeth by 10 months. Once we stopped giving her antibiotics and changed her diet we saw an immediate improvement. Every time she got a tooth over the next eighteen months she would get croup, a stuffy or runny nose and a lot of phlegm. She would also experience a little fever sometimes with irritability. Once she had all of her teeth, she stopped getting sick. She is 3-years-old now and very healthy.

Jack (7 months)
When Jack was three months old he got his two front bottom teeth. He was wakeful, wanting to nurse every few hours, drooled constantly and was

very active. He also made this weird sound, like an old-fashioned electric coffee pot. But then he didn't get any more teeth until he was 7 months, at which point his nose was very congested with mucus and he didn't want to nurse much. He was really cranky and gassy, had trouble sleeping, only took ten minute naps and was very restless at night. It looks like there is another tooth getting ready to come in. He also has nasal congestion and isn't eating very much.

Connor (3 years)
When Connor was teething, he would have watery diarrhea with tummy aches, a stuffy nose and usually a cough. He had all his baby teeth by two years of age, along with eight cavities.

Nicole (2-11 years)
We first took Nicole to Kathy when she was two years old and in the process of getting her two-year molars. She had been on antibiotics continuously from the age of five months for repeated ear and sinus infections. Sleeping was difficult due to bad dreams and she was cranky all the time. She would also have terrible temper tantrums daily. Once Kathy taught us how to rebuild Nicole's immune system and her molars finished coming in, she remained healthy until she started to lose her first baby tooth.

At the age of seven, she had four permanent teeth in front and four loose ones. During that time she started having breathing problems where she felt like she couldn't get air into her lungs, sporadic ear pain, coughs, mucus in the nose, a lot of saliva, sore throats and nightmares. She also started talking back, when ordinarily she was very sweet and responsive. Nicole is now 11 years old and still teething like crazy.

Alexandra (10-16 years)
We first met Kathy when Alex was 10 years old and getting sick all the time. Her nose was very stuffy and she was coughing up mucus. She had a sore throat, a dull ache in her forehead and cheeks and pretty consistent stomach pain. Alex had braces on her teeth that had recently been tightened which coincided with the symptoms.

Kathy explained how braces affect the cranium and that tightening the wires may have contributed to Alex's symptoms. Her advice was to get a chiropractic adjustment to help relieve the stress in her head and suggested the homeopathic remedy Arnica to address any inflammation or pain. We did just that and there was immediate improvement.

The next time I called Kathy, Alex was experiencing: a mild stuffy nose, bad breath, a stomach ache, a subnormal temperature, swollen glands that were worse on the right side, nausea and she was a bit clingy. Kathy reminded me that Alex had once again been to the orthodontist in the days prior to the onset of these physical problems.

The next time Alex had her braces tightened, the same problems occurred, which confirmed a definite connection between the two. The best plan of action for breaking this pattern was to schedule a chiropractic adjustment for the same day as her orthodontist appointment to minimize the repercussions, as well as taking the homeopathic remedy Arnica. This worked well in helping Alex's body adjust.

The only other problem we encountered with Alex's teeth was her eyeteeth did not grow in – there was virtually no sign of them at the age of 15. Consequently, we worked with different homeopathic remedies for nine months to encourage their eruption naturally. Fortunately, one of them did come in on it's own, but the other one needed to be helped along. That's when Alex had surgery to open up the gum and a device was attached to the tooth to encourage its downward movement. The surgery was a complete success and the tooth moved into place within a month and a half. Alex is 16 years old now and there is still no sign of her 12-year molars.

Samantha (infancy-10 years)
When Sami was an infant, we were in a car accident. The car seat flew forward with her in it and her mouth hit the gearshift. Her mouth was bleeding and badly bruised. When her three top front teeth came in on the left side they were deformed, almost like they had been eaten away and discolored. When she was 2-years old and her molars were coming in, something strange happened – her eyes became crossed. Sami's appearance was obviously affected by both of these events and she went through her early years with other kids always teasing her and low self-esteem. My

personal theory about the situation is that the accident, teeth and eyes were in some way connected. No medical physician has ever confirmed this thought.

Samantha is a very healthy child. She is never sick and always has a good appetite. As she grew up and her teeth became loose, I noticed that with the movement of each tooth she would get a cold or flu and her appetite would disappear. My personal experience in observing Sami's teething process has shown me that she does experience a weaker immune system with the loss or eruption of each tooth. Out of the three teeth that were affected by the accident – the front tooth did come in deformed and needed to be capped; the one next to it was okay and her eyetooth has not yet erupted, so we will just have to wait and see.

Rebecca (5 years)
When Rebecca was five and a half and started cutting her 6-year molars, she experienced cold like symptoms with a green, runny, drippy nose. We tried natural methods to cure the infection with no results. Eventually, she was given two rounds of antibiotics (approximately 20 days) but they didn't help either.

Finally, I called Kathy and told her what was going on with Rebecca. Her first question was, "Is she getting her 6-year molars?" Rebecca opened her mouth and sure enough, her two top molars were just breaking through the gum. Her sinus condition was persistent for several months until the molars were about halfway in, at which point all the nasal congestion cleared up on its own. She did not experience the same condition with the bottom molars, but she did have a cough.

Jake (20 months)
When Jake was 20 months old, we were on the road traveling when he got a severe case of croup. He was ordinarily a healthy baby and had only experienced croup one other time in his life. He was also extremely fussy which was out of character. One of my dear friends suggested I call Kathy and perhaps she would be able to help. Once we established Jake's age, she suggested that teething might be the reason for his symptoms. So I looked in his mouth and sure enough he was getting two of his molars. When I

thought back, I realized the last time he had croup was about a year ago, when he was getting his first molars.

Billy (16 years)

Around the time of Billy's 16th birthday, he complained of a headache, sore throat and earache. It was the third time in the past two months he'd experienced the same type of symptoms. As Billy revealed other symptoms (i.e. ear and throat pain, mood swings, headaches, nasal congestion and gas) to us, Kathy jokingly asked him if he had any teeth coming in. To all our surprise, he said, yes, his upper left wisdom tooth was just breaking through. Billy had gotten his 12-year molars at 14, so we never expected his wisdom teeth to be coming in at 16 – Happy birthday Billy!

Conclusion

Perhaps these stories will give you greater insight in understanding the teething process in relation to your child's physical, emotional and behavioral problems. There will be times when teething is the underlying cause of a child's problems, and other times when a child is actually sick, reacting to an environmental or food allergy, hormonal disturbance, mimicking learned behaviors, or experiencing family or social trauma. My hope is that this book will increase parents' awareness of the contributing factors to a problem and give then the courage and tools to address the issues from a different perspective. Never assume that a symptom is the result of teething. Always, thoroughly evaluate the situation and consult with a medical professional regarding all health related issues.

Notes

Chapter one

1. Theodore Berland & Alfred Seyler, *Your Children's Teeth*, Meredith Press, 1968; 10-11.

2. Schafer, Elizabeth, *Eat Wisely For You & Your Baby*, February 12, 1995.

3. Walter T. McFall Jr., "Oral Histology," *Dental Assistant* - Chapter 5; 107-108.

4. Stay, Flora Parsa, D.D.S., *The Complete Book of Dental Remedies*, Avery Publishing Group, 1996; 8.

5. Walter T. McFall Jr., "Oral Histology," *Dental Assistant* - Chapter 5; 107-108.

6. R. Jack Shankle, "Dental Anatomy & Physiology," *Dental Assistant* - Chapter 4; 90.

7. Walter T. McFall Jr., "Oral Histology," *Dental Assistant* - Chapter 5; 109.

8. Ibid.; 108-112.

9. Zand, Walton, Rountree, *Smart Medicine For A Healthier Child*, Avery Publishing Group, 1994; 44.

10. Moll, Lucy, *The Vegetarian Child - A Complete Guide for Parents*, Perigee/Parenting Health, 1997; 16-17.

11. "Fats: Facts & Fiction," *Omega Nutrition Product Book*, (since 1987), 1998 copy; 4.

12. Hibbeln JR., Seafood consumption, the DHA content of mother's milk and prevalence rates of postpartum depression: *Journal of Affective Disorders 2001*.

13. Levenstein, Barbara M.S. Nutrition "How to Tell A Good Fat From A Bad One," *Creative Health Newsletter,* 1999/Winter; 10.

14. Galland, Leo M.D., *Superimmunity For Kids*, A Copestone Press (Dell Trade Paperback), 1989; XIX, 7-9.

15. The Burton Goldberg Group, *Alternative Medicine - The Definitive Guide*, Future Medicine Publishing, 1993; 167.

16. Balch M.D., James & Balch C.N.C., Phyllis, *Prescription for Nutritional Healing*, Avery, 1990; 12.

17. Eisenberg, Murkoff & Hathaway, *What To Expect When You're Expecting*, Workman Publishing Co., 1996.

18. Schoelen, Charles (Nutritionist), "Minerals The Building Blocks of the Body," *New Editions Health Word*; 20-21.

19. Sacks, Adam D., "Weston Price - Quest for The Healthy Tooth," *Mothering Magazine, Fall* – 1984; 29-30.

20. Albrecht M.S., C.N., Frances, "Are You Getting Enough Calcium?" *Delicious Magazine*, September 1996; 36.

21. Ibid.

22. Nash, Francesca & Roberts, Janette, *Healthy Parents, Better Babies*, The Crossing Press, 1999; 43.

23. Galland, Leo M.D., *Superimmunity For Kids*, A Copestone Press (Dell Trade Paperback), 1989; 38-39.

24. Charles Attwood M.D., F.A.A.P., *Dr. Attwood's Lowfat Prescription for Kids*, Penguim Group, N.Y., 1996; 66.

25. Lovendale, Mark, "Your Health and Dairy Products," *Mother to Mother; Another View*; No. 22, 1993.

26. Jarrow Formulas Inc. "A Statement About Calcium Supplements & Lead," *Press Release*, March 24, 1997; 8.
27. "Baby Needs Calcium," *L.A. Parent Magazine*, 1998; 30.
28. Oski M.D., Frank A., *Don't Drink Your Milk!* Teach Services, Inc, Ninth Edition, 1995; 4-5.
29. Ibid.
30. Ibid.; 48.
31. Lovendale, Mark, "Your Health and Dairy Products," *Mother to Mother; Another View*; No. 22, 1993; 4.
32. *Food Values of Portions Commonly Used*, Pennington JAT Bowes & Church's Harper & Row 1989.
33. O'Mara, Peggy, *Natural Family Living,* Pocket Book, A division of Simon & Schuster, Inc., March 2000; 139-140.
34. Romm, Aviva Jill, *The Natural Pregnancy Book*, The Crossing Press; 1997; 55-56.
35. Hudson N.D., Tori, *Womans Encyclopedia of Natural Medicine*, Keats, 1999; 230-231.
36. Balch M.D., James & Balch C.N.C., Phyllis, *Prescription for Nutritional Healing,* Avery, 1990; 18.
37. Hudson N.D., Tori, *Womans Encyclopedia of Natural Medicine*, Keats, 1999; 229-231.
38. Nash, Francesca & Roberts, Janette, *Healthy Parents, Better Babies*, The Crossing Press, 1999; 37-39.
39. Ibid.
40. Ibid.; 41.
41. Romm, Aviva Jill, *The Natural Pregnancy Book*, The Crossing Press; 1997; 52-53.
42. Nash, Francesca & Roberts, Janette, *Healthy Parents, Better Babies*, The Crossing Press, 1999; 47.
43. Hudson N.D., Tori, *Womans Encyclopedia of Natural Medicine*, Keats, 1999; 229.
44. Marilyn J. Bush & A.J. Verlangieri, "An acute study on the relative gastro intestinal absorption of a noval form of calcium ascorbate," Antherosclerosis Research Laboratories, Dept of Pharmacology, School of Pharmacy, University of Mississippi - Excerpts from *Research Communications in Chemical Pathology & Pharmacology*, Vol. 57, No1, 1987.
45. Romm, Aviva Jill, *The Natural Pregnancy Book*, The Crossing Press; 1997; 54-55.
46. O'Mara, Peggy, *Natural Family Living*, Pocket Book, A division of Simon & Schuster, Inc., March 2000; 123.
47. Galland, Leo M.D., *Superimmunity For Kids,* A Copestone Press (Dell Trade Paperback), 1989; 75.
48. O'Mara, Peggy, *Natural Family Living*, Pocket Book, A division of Simon & Schuster, Inc., March 2000; 125-128.236
49. Galland, Leo M.D., *Superimmunity For Kids*, A Copestone Press (Dell Trade Paperback), 1989; 76.
50. Susan Roberts Ph.D., Melvin Hayman, M.D., Lisa Tracy, *Feeding Your Child For Lifelong Health*, Bantam Books, 1999; 144.
51. Ibid. 36-37.
52. Charles Attwood M.D., F.A.A.P., *Dr. Attwood's Lowfat Prescription for Kids*, Penguim Group, N.Y., 1996; 62-64.

53. Oski M.D., Frank A., *Don't Drink Your Milk!* Teach Services, Inc, Ninth Edition, 1995; 16-18.

54. Hal Huggins, D.D.S.,M.S. *Why Raise Ugly Kids*, Crown, NY, 1981; 87-88.

55. Balch M.D., James & Balch C.N.C., Phyllis, *Prescription for Nutritional Healing*, Avery, 1990; 18, 227.

Chapter two

1. Theodore Berland & Alfred Seyler D.D.S., *Your Children's Teeth*, Meredith Press, 1968; 30-31.

2. Formur Inc., *Biochemic Handbook*, 1976; 67-68, 100 – originally published as Biochemic Theory & Practice, by J.B. Chapman, M.D. & Edward L. Perry, M.D.

3. Theodore Berland & Alfred Seyler D.D.S., *Your Children's Teeth*, Meredith Press, 1968; 30-31.

4. Bernard Lievegoed, *Phases of Childhood*, Floris Books – Anthroposophic Press; 1987; 23-24.

Chapter three

1. Marvin S. Eiger, M.D. & Sally Wendkos Olds, *The Complete Book of Breastfeeding*, 3rd edition, 1999; 6-7.

2. Ibid.; 6-7.

3. "Pediatrics," *American Academy of Pediatrics*, (AAP) Volume 100, No 6, December 1997; 1035-1039.

4. Theodore Berland & Alfred Seyler, D.D.S., *Your Children's Teeth*, Meredith Press, N.Y., 1968; 16-18.

5. Kathy Arnos, Phone interview with Marc Harmon, D.D.S., December 1999.

6. Marvin S. Eiger, M.D. & Sally Wendkos Olds, *The Complete Book of Breastfeeding*, 3rd edition, 1999; 16-17.

7. Donald Getz, O.D., F.A.A.O., F.C.O.V.D., "Understanding Your Child's Visual Wellness," *Mother to Mother; Another View*, December 1992; 8-9.

8. "Pediatrics," *American Academy of Pediatrics*; 1035-1039.

9. Marvin S. Eiger, M.D. & Sally Wendkos Olds, *The Complete Book of Breastfeeding*, 3rd edition, 1999; 1-2.

10. Ibid.; 62-63.

11. Ruth Lawrence, "Biochemistry of Human Milk," *Breastfeeding – A Guide for the Medical Profession*, 4th edition, Mosby Year Book, 1994; 95.

12. Dr. Daniel Clark, "The Colostrum Miracle – Too Good to Be True," *Vital Health News*, Winter 1998; 1,13.

13. Wendy Block, "The French Secret to Long Healthy Life," *Creative Health Newsletter*, Summer 1998; 1-2.

14. Ibid.

15. Maureen Minchin, "What Is Wrong With Infant Formula?" *Mother to Mother; Another View*, April/May 1990; 14-15.

16. Bonnie Liebman, "Baby Formula; Missing Key Facts?," *CCL Family Foundations*, July/Aug 1991; 14-15.

17. Marvin S. Eiger, M.D. & Sally Wendkos Olds, *The Complete Book of Breastfeeding*, 3rd edition, 1999; 7-8.

18. Ruth Lawrence, "Biochemistry of Human Milk," *Breastfeeding – A Guide for the*

Medical Profession, 4th edition, Mosby Year Book, 1994; 149-179.

19. Marvin S. Eiger, M.D. & Sally Wendkos Olds, *The Complete Book of Breastfeeding*, 3rd edition, 1999; 9-13.

20. Maureen Minchin, "What Is Wrong With Infant Formula?" *Mother to Mother; Another View*, April/May 1990; 14-15.

21. Ibid.

22. Susan B. Roberts, Ph.D., Melvin Heyman, M.D., & LisaTracy, *Feeding Your Child for Lifelong Health*, A Bantam Book, 1999; 90.

23. Michelle Badash, "DHA's Role in Infant Development," *Nutrition Science News*, April 1997; 196-197.

24. Leo Galland, M.D. & Dian Dincin Buchman, Ph.D., *Superimmunity, Dell Publishing*, 1989; 67.

25. Susan B. Roberts, Ph.D., Melvin Heyman, M.D., & LisaTracy, *Feeding Your Child for Lifelong Health*, A Bantam Book, 1999; 90.

26. Sara Ani, "Breastfeeding and Dental Caries," *Mothering Magazine*, Fall 1986; 29.

27. Rosemarie Van Norman, *Helping The Thumb-sucking Child*, Avery, 1999; XI-XII.

28. Ibid.

29. Ibid.

30. Theodore Berland & Alfred Seyler, D.D.S., *Your Children's Teeth*, Meredith Press, N.Y., 1968; 21.

31. Rosemarie Van Norman, *Helping The Thumb-sucking Child*, Avery, 1999; 10.

32. Ibid.; 20-25, 28, 45.

33. Ibid.; 11-12.

34. Ibid.

35. Kathy Arnos, Phone interview with Marc Harmon, D.D.S., December 1999.

36. Ibid.

Chapter four

1. Janet Zand LAc., OMD, Rachel Walton, RN, Bob Rountree, M.D., *Smart Medicine for A Healthier Child*, Avery Publishing Group, NY, 1994; 234-235.

2. L Jarber; IJ Cohen; A Mor, "Arch Dis Child," Sambur Centre of Pediatric Hematology/oncology, Beilinson Medical Centre, Sackler School of Medicine Tel Aviv University, February 1992; 233-234.

3. Janet Zand LAc., OMD, Rachel Walton, RN, Bob Rountree, M.D., *Smart Medicine for A Healthier Child*, Avery Publishing Group, NY, 1994; 236.

4. Michael Schmidt, Lendon Smith, M.D., Keith Sehnert, *Beyond Antibiotics*, North Atlantic Books 1993; 245.

5. Michael Schmidt, *Childhood Ear Infections - What Every Parent & Physician Should Know*, North Atlantic Books 1990; 3-8.

6. Ibid.

7. Lynne Paige Walker DOP, Ellen Hodgson Brown, *The Informed Consumer's Pharmacy*, Carroll & Graf Publishers, Inc. NY, 1990; 43-46.

8. Michael Schmidt, *Childhood Ear Infections - What Every Parent & Physician Should Know*, North Atlantic Books 1990; 21-26.

9. Valerie Ann Worwood, *The Complete Book of Essential Oils & Aromatherapy*, New World Library, 1991; 31-32.

10. Roberta Wilson, *A Complete Guide to Understanding & Using Aromatherapy For Vibrant Health & Beauty*, Avery, 1994; 123-124.
11. Dr. James & Phyllis Balch, *Prescription for Nutritional Healing*, Avery Publishing Group 1990;115.
12. Jane Hersey, *Why Can't My Child Behave?*, Pear Tree Press, Inc., 1996;19-20.
13. DL King; W. Steinhauer; Garcia-Godoy; CJ Elkins, "Herpetic Gingivostomatitis & Teething Difficulty in Infants," *University of Texas Health Science Center in San Antonio*, (Pediatric Dept.), Mar-April 1992; 82-85.
14. Kathy Arnos, "Coxsackie A Mini Epidemic," *Mother to Mother; Another View*; Oct/Nov 1990;12.
15. Ibid.
16. Kelly Patricia O'Meara, "Doping Kids," *Insight, A Publication of The Washington Times Corp.*, June 28, 1999; 11.
17. Ibid.;11.
18. Ibid. And Judith Reichenberg-Ullman N.D., MSW, & Robert Ullman, N.D., *Ritalin Free Kids*, Prima Publishing 1996; 40.
19. Ibid Judith Reichenberg-Ullman N.D., MSW, & Robert Ullman, N.D., 1996; XV.
20. Kelly Patricia O'Meara, "Doping Kids," *Insight, A Publication of The Washington Times Corp.*, June 28, 1999;12.
21. Bruce Wiseman, "Psychiatry & The Creation of Senseless Violence," *Citizens Commission on Human Rights Int.*, May 1999; 6-8.
22. Depositions supplied by Michael O'Brien, Director of Public Information for The Citizens Commission on Human Rights,1990.
23. Bruce Wiseman, "Psychiatry & The Creation of Senseless Violence," *Citizens Commission on Human Rights Int.*, May 1999; 6.
24. Ibid.; 8; and 20/20 Barbara Walters Interum with Strokmeyer, July 9, 1999, 10:00p.m.

Chapter five
1. Hathaway, Hargreaves, Thompson, Novitsky, "A Study into the Effects of Light on Children of Elementary School Age – A Case of Daylight Robbery," *Alberta Education*, February 1992.
2. Stephen J. Moss, *Your Child's Teeth: A Parent's Guide to Making and Keeping Them Perfect* (Boston: Houghton Mifflin Company, 1977); 4, 10-11.
3. Ibid.; 5.
4. David C. Johnsen, "Dental Caries Patterns in Preschool Children," *Dent.Clin. North Am.*, volume 28, no. 1 (January 1984); 9.
5. F. Batmanghelidj, M.D., *Your Body's Many Cries for Water – You Are Not Sick*, Global Health Solutions Inc., 1995; 15.
6. Sara Ani, "Breastfeeding and Dental Caries," *Mothering Magazine*, Fall 1986: 29-37.
7. Ibid.; 31-32.
8. Winifred G. Hammond, *The Riddle of Teeth*, Coward, McCann & Geoghegan, 1971; 39-40.
9. Hal Huggins, *Why Raise Ugly Kids?*, Crown, N.Y.,1981; 142-146.
10. George E. Meinig, D.D.S., F.A.C.D., "What Chewing Gum Manufacturers Don't Want You To Know," *Mother to Mother: Another View*, Fall 1991; 9, 22.

11. Ibid.

12. Stephen J. Moss, Your Child's *Teeth: A Parent's Guide to Making and Keeping Them Perfect*, Boston: Houghton Mifflin Company, 1977; 4.

13. Ibid.; 78-79.

14. Barry K. Chudakov, "Sugar in Medications: The Covert Contributor to Dental Disease," *Journal of the Canadian Dental Association*, Volume 50, No. 8 (August 1984); 613.

15. W.J. Loesche, "Nutrition and Dental Decay in Infants," *American Journal of Clinical Nutrition*, Volume 41 (February 1985); 423, 425-428.

16. Hal Huggins, *Why Raise Ugly Kids?*, Crown, N.Y.,1981;142-146.

17. Theodore Berland, Alfred Seyler, D.D.S., *Your Children's Teeth*, Meredith Press, 1968; 9-14.

18. Benjamin Spock M.D. & Michael B. Rothenberg M.D., *Dr. Spock's Baby and Child Care*, Sixth Edition, Duttan, 1992; 323-324.

19. George E. Meinig, *Root Canal Cover-up*, Fourth Printing, Bion, Ojai, CA., 1996;140-141.

20. Ibid.; VI.

21. Ibid.; VI-VII, 25.

22. Ibid.; 1-6.

23. Weiss, B; Landrigan, PJ. "The Developing Brain and the Environment, An Introduction." *Environmental Health Perspective*, June, 108(3); 373-4.

24. Richard Casdorph, M.D., Morton Walker, D.P.M., *Toxic Metal Syndrome*, Avery, 1995; 148.

Chapter six

1. John Yiamouyiannis, *Fluoride: the Aging Factor*, Third edition, Health Action Press, 1993; 13.

2. Ibid.; 7-25.

3. "Caries, Diagnosis & Risk Assessment," *American Dental Association Publishing Company*, June 1995; 19F.

4. Frank Murray, *The Big Family Guide toThe Minerals,* Keats, 1995; 281-282.

5. Lynn Landes & Maria Bechis, "America Overdosed on Fluoride", *Zero Waste America*, updated 1998; 1-2.

6. "A Strange Little Secret About Fluoride Supplementation", *Pure Facts*, A Newsletter for the Feingold Association, April 2001.

7. Ibid.

8. John Yiamouyiannis, *Fluoride: the Aging Factor*, Third edition, Health Action Press, 1993; 40-41.

9. Ibid.; 34-39.

10. Ibid.; 4.

11. Ibid.

12. Ibid.; 41-46.

13. Frank Murray, *The Big Family Guide to The Minerals*, Keats, 1995; 298.

14. Ibid.; 290.

15. John Yiamouyiannis, *Fluoride: the Aging Factor*, Third edition, Health Action Press, 1993; 134-135.

16. Thomas McGuire, D.D.S., *Tooth Fitness*, St. Michaels Press, 1994; 302-304.

17. Lynn Landes & Maria Bechis, "America Overdosed on Fluoride", *Zero Waste America*, updated 1998; 1-2.

18. John Yiamouyiannis, *Fluoride: the Aging Factor*, Third edition, *Health Action Press*, 1993; 62-71.

19. Joel Griffiths & Chris Bryson, "Fluoride, Teeth and the A-Bomb,"*Earth Island Journal*, Winter 1997-98; 38-41.

20. Safe Water Coalition of Washington State, "Fluoride Has Adverse Effect on Central Nervous System," *Townsend Letter for Doctors & Patients*, June 1996; 21.

21. Editorial by AWB & JC, "Neurotoxicity of Fluoride,"*Fluoride Journal*, November 1996; 29: 2, 57-58.

22. LiXS, Zhi JL, Gao RO, "Effect of Fluoride Exposure on Intelligence in Children,"*Fluoride Journal,* November 1995; 28:4; 189-192.

23. Vincent Kierman, "Chemical in Fluoridated Water May Cause Violent Behavior & Cocaine Use,"*Academe Today*, September 8, 1998.

24. Frank Murray, *The Big Family Guide to The Minerals*, Keats, 1995; 285.

25. John Yiamouyiannis, *Fluoride: the Aging Factor*, Third edition, Health Action Press, 1993; 14.

26. Ibid.; 13-14.

27. D. Kennedy D.D.S., "Questions & Answers", *Preventive Dental Health Association and Sizzle!* Productions, http://emporium.turnpike.net/P/PDHA/health.htm

28. Ibid.; 17-19.

29. Frank Murray, *The Big Family Guide toThe Minerals*, Keats, 1995; 300-301.

30. John Yiamouyiannis, *Fluoride: the Aging Factor*, Third edition, Health Action Press, 1993; 105.

31. Thomas McGuire, D.D.S., *Tooth Fitness*, St. Michaels Press, 1994; 298.

32. Lynn Landes & Maria Bechis, "America Overdosed on Fluoride", *Zero Waste America*, updated 1998; 1-2.

Chapter seven

1. *Physicians Desk Reference for Nonprescription Drugs*, 17th edition, 1996; 667.

2. Kathy Arnos, phone interview, Rose Ann Soloway, an administrator at The American Association of Poison Control Center in Washington, D.C., 1997.

3. Thomas McGuire, D.D.S., *Tooth Fitness*, St. Michael's Press, 1994; 98.

4. "Adverse Effects of 'Inactive' Ingredients", The American Academy of Pediatrics Committee on Drugs, *Pediatrics*, October 1985 and Public Citizen Health Research Group, *Health Letter*, March/April 1985.

5. Winstron & Williams, *Journal American Dietetic Association* 1997; 532-534.

6. "Saccharin", *Journal American Dietetic Association* 1998; 98, 580-587.

7. John Yiamouyiannis, *Fluoride: The Aging Factor*, Third edition, Health Action Press, 1993;14.

8. Bausch & Lomb, *Health Watch*, June 1993.

9. "Adverse Effects of 'Inactive' Ingredients", The American Academy of Pediatrics Committee on Drugs, *Pediatrics*, October 1985 and Public Citizen Health Research Group, *Health Letter*, March/April 1985.

10. Jane Hersey, *Why Can't My Child Behave*, Pear Tree Press, 1996; 65-72.

11. Lisa Y. Lefferts, MSPH, "Toxic Dentistry – Nothing to Smile About",

The Green Guide, #30, October 1996; 1-3.

12. "Many Ways to Disrupt the Hormone System – New Toxicological Patterns", Birnbaum, L.S. 1994; Colborn, T. & C. Clement, 1992; Colborn, T. 1994; Colborn, T., D. Dumanoski & P. Myers, 1996; Kelse et al, 1995; Luoma, J.R., 1995; Mably et al, 1991; Soto, A.M. et al, 1991; Soto, A.M., et al, 1994.

13. Lisa Y. Lefferts, MSPH, "Toxic Dentistry – Nothing to Smile About", *The Green Guide*, #30, October 1996;1-3.

14. "Plastics Makers Ordered to Recall Tableware", *Mainichi Daily News*, April 15, 1998; 12.

15. Lisa Y. Lefferts, MSPH, "Toxic Dentistry – Nothing to Smile About", *The Green Guide*, #30, October 1996; 1-3.

16. Tricia Toyota, Channel 2, "Evening News – Consumer Reports," Los Angeles, May 1999.

17. "Parents May Want to Replace Some Baby Bottles and Teething," *Consumer Reports*, May 1999.

18. Ibid.

19. Ibid.

20. Ibid.

21. Frank Jerome, D.D.S., *Tooth Truth*, Promotion Publishing, 1995; 94-97.

22. A. O. Summers, J. Wireman, M.J. Vimy, F.L. Lorscheider, B. Marshall, S.B. Levy, S. Bennett, and L. Billard, "Mercury Released form Dental "Silver" Fillings Provokes an Increase in Mercury and Antibiotic-Resistant Bacteria in Oral & Intestinal Floras of Primates", Antimicrobial Agents and Chemotherapy, April 1993; 825-834.

23. Frank Jerome, D.D.S., *Tooth Truth*, Promotion Publishing, 1995; 94-96.

24. Vicki Mabrey, "60 Minutes II" (transcripts), Dentist & Children, January 20, 1999; 9.

25. Ibid: 10.

26. Ibid: 11.

27. Lita Lee, Ph.D., *Radiation Protection Manuel,* Third edition, 1990; 17-24.

28. Flora Parsa Stay, D.D.S., *The Complete Book of Dental Remedies*, Avery, 1995; 160-161.

29. Ibid.

30. Kim Laurell, D.D.S., M.S., "Diagnosis of Erosion Due to Bulemia & Other Acids", 1999: http://www.prosthinfo.com.

31. Flora Parsa Stay, D.D.S., *The Complete Book of Dental Remedies*, Avery, 1995; 155-156.

32. Barry Skaggs, D.D.S., "Coping with Baby's Dental Emergencies", *Wet Set Gazette*, September 1993; 2, 14.

33. Scientific Basis for Save-A-Tooth

34. *Press Release Phoenix-Lazerus, Inc.* – New State of Ohio order Mandates All Child-care Facilities to Have First-aid Items to Save Knocked-out Teeth – 2003.

35. Paul Krasner D.D.S., "A New Philosophy For The Treatment of Avulsed Teeth", *Journal of Oral Surgery, Oral Medicine and Oral Pathology*, 1995; 79: 616-623.

36. Ibid.

37. Flora Parsa Stay, D.D.S., *The Complete Book of Dental Remedies*, Avery, 1995; 175.

38. Theodore Berland & Alfred Seyler, *Your Children's Teeth*, Meredith Press, N.Y., 1968; 111.

Chapter eight

1. Mr. Randal Helliot, "Examination of Bristle Tip Geometry and Fixing of the Bristles in a Toothbrush With Replaceable Heads," Report issued by J. Hilary Holgate/Jill Webb, *Microscopy Laboratory*, Oct. 17, 1997; 5.

2. Marc Warsowe, News Release, "Terradent Replaceable Head Toothbrush Introduced," Eco-DenT International, Redwood City, CA; 1998.

3. Richard L. Meckstroth, D.D.S., "Improving Quality and Efficiency in Oral Hygiene," *Journal of Gerontological Nursing* Vol. 15, No. 6; 38.

4. Karen D. Avey, BS, "Give Your Teeth a Hug: A Simplified Brushing Technique for Children," *Journal of Dentistry for Children*, Sept.-Oct. 1984; 371-373.

5. Peter P. Kambjy, D.D.S., MS, Steven M. Levy, D.D.S., MPH, "An Evaluation of the Effectiveness of Four Mechanical Plaque-removal Devices When Used by a Trained Care-provider", *Special Care in Dentistry*, Vol. 13, No. 1, 1993; 12.

6. Naseeb Shory, D.D.S., MPH, George Mitchell, D.M.D.,MPH, Homer Jamison, D.D.S., Dr Ph, "A Study of the Effectiveness of Two Types of Toothbrushes for Removal of Oral Accumulations", *JADA*, Vol. 115, Nov. 19, 1987; 717-720.

7. Eli Grossman, D.D.S.; Howard Proskin, Ph.D., "A Comparison of The Efficacy & Safety of an Electric & A Manual Children's Toothbrush," *JADA*, Vol. 128, April 1997; 469-474.

8. Ibid.

9. R.L. Boyd, P. Murray, "Effect of Rotary Electric Toothbrush versus Manuel Toothbrush on Periodontal Status During Orthodontic Treatment", *American Journal of Orthodontics and Dentofacial Surgery*, 1989; Vol. 96, No. 4, 342-347.

10. Larry W. White, D.D.S., M.S.D., "Efficacy of a Sonic Toothbrush in Reducing Plaque and Gingivitis in Adolescent Patients", *Journal of Clinical Orthodontics*, February 1996; Vol. XXX, No. 2.

11. Ha Phan Ho, Richard Niederman, "Effectiveness of the Sonicare Sonic Toothbrush on Reduction of Plaque, Gingivitis, Probing Pocket Depth and Subgingival Bacteria in Adolescent Orthodontic Patients", *Journal of Clinical Dentistry*, 1997, Vo. VIII, No. 1, 15-18.

12. Flora Parsa Stay, D.D.S., *The Complete Book of Dental Remedies*, Avery Publishing Group, 1996; 178-179.

13. Sabine Gerasch, "Children-Toothbrushes," (*Consumer Reports* in Frankfurt, German) *OKO-Test Magazine*, Issue 6, June; 1998.

14. Ibid.

15. Thomas McGuire, D.D.S., *Tooth Fitness*: Your Guide to Healthy Teeth, St Michael's Press, 1994; 287-288.

16. Gilmoe EL, Gross A, Whiteley R. "Effect of Tongue Brushing on Plaque Bacteria," *Oral Surgery*, 1973; 36, 201-204.

17. Jacobson SE, Crawford JJ, McFall WR., "Oral Physiotherapy of the Tongue and Palate: Relationship to Plaque Control," *Journal of the American Dental Association*, 1973; 87, 134-139.

18. Tom's of Maine Product & Ingredient Fact Sheet on Fluoride, 1998.

19. J. Gultz, D.D.S.; L. Do, B.S.; W. Scherer, D.D.S., abstract "The Antimicrobial Activity Produced by Five Commercially Available Dentifrices," *New York University College of Dentistry*, October, 1997.

20. D. Estafan, D.D.S.; J.Gultz, D.D.S.; J.M. Kaim, D.D.S.; Khaghany, B.S.;W.Scherer, D.D.S., "Clinical Efficacy of an Herbal Toothpaste," The *Journal of Clinical Dentistry*, 1998;Vol. IX, No. 2; 31-33.

21. William A. Saupe, D.D.S., "The Effect of Various Dentifrices on Demineralized Human Tooth Enamel In Vitro," Abrasivity of Four Commercially Available Dentifrices, *UCSF*, 1991; 1-14.

22. Ibid.

23. Jennifer C. Davis, "Something to Smile About," *Delicious! Magazine*, February 1997: 52.

24. Ibid.

25. J. Gultz, D.D.S., L.Do, B.S., J.Kaim, D.D.S., W.Scherer, D.D.S., "Antimicrobial Activity of an Herbal Mouth rinse," "An In Vitro Investigation of the Antimicrobial Activity of an Herbal Mouth rinse," *The Journal of Clinical Dentistry*, 1998;Vol.IX, No. 2, *New York University College of Dentistry*, Abstract 1998; 3, (212) 998-9426.

26. Peelu The Natural Toothcare Company, "An Ancient Secret to Whiter Teeth and Healthier Gums," *Press Release*.

27. Kurt Cameron, "Brushing Up On Prevention – An Interview With a Holistic Dentist,"; 94-95.

28. Marc Warsowe, *News Release* "Between! Natural Baking Soda Dental Gum Launched!," Eco-Dent International.

29. K.K. Makinen, P.L. Makinen, H.R. Pape, Jr., P.Allen, C.A. Bennett, P.J. Isokangas, K.P. Isotupa, "Xylitol and Its Effect on Dental Caries," *International Dental Journal*, February 1995; Vol. 45, No.1 (Supplement 1); 93-107.

30. David Richard, *Stevia Rebaudiana, Nature's Sweet Secret*, Vital Health Publishing, 2nd edition – 1998; 19.

31. Donna Gates, L. Bonvie, B. Bonvie, *The Stevia Story - A Tale of Incredible Sweetness and Intrigue*, B.E.D. Publications Co., 1997; 25-26, 53-54.

Chapter nine

1. N. Rowan Richards D.C., "Inside the Problem Child," *Mother to Mother: Another View*, Dec/Jan 1990; 4-7.

2. N. Rowan Richards D.C.; "The Relationship of Teething and The Cranium", Phone interview by Kathy Arnos, Van Nuys, CA, 1993.

3. John Upledger, D.O., FAAO, "The relationship of craniosacral examination findings in grade school children with developmental problems," *Journal AOA*, Vol. 77, June 1976.

4. Hal Huggins, D.D.S.,M.S. *Why Raise Ugly Kids*, Crown, NY, 1981; 6.

5. Ibid.

6. Ibid.; 9.

7. Ibid.; 29-52.

8. Ibid.

9. Ibid.; 88.

10. Ibid.; 87-88.

11. Frank Jerome D.D.S., *Tooth Truth*, Promotion Publishing, 1995; 297-298.

12. Marc Harmon D.D.S., "Crozat Therapy – How You Can Shape Your Child's Face," *Mother to Mother: Another View*, No. 20, 1992; 8.

13. Ibid.

Resource Guide

Oral Care

Collis Curve Toothbrush, Inc.
www.colliscurve.com
800-298-4818
Unique dentist developed tooth-brush.

Eco-DenT International
www.eco-dent.com
800-369-6933
Oral care products; Terradent replaceable head toothbrush, kids & adults.

Gillette Company
www.oralb.com
Kids Oral-B stages, manual tooth-brushes/Kids Power Toothbrush.

HoMedics, Inc.
www.homedics.com
Electric toothbrushes

IMHOTEP, Inc.
See herb section.

Jason
www.jason-natural.com
877-527-6601
Natural cosmetics & oral care products.

Nature's Answer
See herb section.

Nature's Gate
www.levlad.com
800-327-2012
Oral & body care products.

Pureline Oralcare
www.purelineoralcare.com
877-662-9500
Homeopathic teething gel, breath gel, plastic tongue cleaner.

Recycline
www.recycline.com
888-354-7296
The Preserve toothbrush – made from recycled materials, comes with recycling mailer; tongue cleaner.

The Natural Dentist
www.thenaturaldentist.com
800-615-6895
Oral care products.

Peelu Company
www.swansonvitamins.com
800-451-3358
Oral care products.

Philips Oral Healthcare
www.sonicare.com
800-676-7664
Sonicare, the Sonic toothbrush.

Phoenix-Lazerus, Inc.
www.save-a-tooth.com
888-788-6684
Save-A-Tooth preserving system.

Pro-Dentec
www.prodentec.com
Available at dental offices
Rota-dent one step electric
toothbrush.

Tom's of Maine
www.tomsofmaine.com
800-367-8667
Oral care products.

Weleda
www.usa.weleda.com
800-241-1030
Oral & body care products, nursing
tea, etc.

Nutritional Products

Barlean's
www.barleans.com
800-445-3529
Essential fatty acids.

ChildLife
www.childlife.net
800-993-0332
Complete nutritional program for
infants and kids.

Country Life
www.country-life.com
800-645-5768
Nutritional supplements all ages,
prenatal vitamin.

Enzymatic Therapy
www.enzy.com
800-783-2286
Kids multi-vitamin & mineral,
concentration & immune formulas.

Fit for You
www.miraclegreens.com
800-521-jump
Complete nutritional powder with
fruits & vegetables.

Health From the Sun
www.healthfromthesun.com
800-447-2249
Essential fatty acids (EFA) all ages,
homeopathic combinations.

Highland Laboratories
www.highlandvitamins.com
888-717-4917
Multi-vitamins, herbal formulas for
respiratory, allergy, ears, throat,
immune system.

Innovative Natural Products
www.inponline.com
800-893-7467
Multi-vitamins & minerals,
concentration formula, colloidal
formulas.

Jarrow Formulas
www.Jarrow.com
800-726-0886
Nutritional supplements all ages,
prenatal vitamin.

Natrol, Inc.
www.natrol.com or
800-326-1520
Kids liquid multi-vitamin, liquid
memory formula, prenatal vitamin.

Natural Factors
www.naturalfactors.com
800-322-8704
Brain, gastrointestinal & immune
support, vitamins, DHA.

Naturally Vitamins
www.naturally.com
800-899-4499
Inuflora – prebiotic for all ages
(intestinal health.)

NF Formulas
www.nfformulas.com
800-547-4891
Liquid calcium & magnesium –
vanilla flavored (equal ratios). Only
available through healthcare practitioners or mail order (See end of
resource list.)

Nutrition Now, Inc.
www.nutritionnow.com
800-9929-0418
Kids multi-vitamin/minerals, herbs.

Rainbow Light
www.rainbowlight.com
800-635-1233
Kids multi-vitamins with herbs and
vegetable extracts, immune formula, prenatal support and vitamins.

Spectrum Essentials
www.spectrumnaturals.com
800-995-2705
Essential fatty acids & fiber.

Super Nutrition
www.supernutrition.com
800-262-2116
Kids multi-vitamin (for child old
enough to swallow small tablets),
prenatal.

Homeopathics & Flower Essences

Aqua Flora
www.aqua-flora.com
800-237-4100
Homeopathic liquid for candida.

Heel Inc.
www.HeelUSA.com
800-621-7644
Combination homeopathic formulas, topicals, sprays, eye drops, etc.

Boiron USA
www.boiron.com
800-258-8823 (blu-tube)
Single homeopathic medicines,

specialty formulas, eye drops, topicals, etc.

Boericke & Tafel, Inc.
www.naturesway.com
800-962-8873
Combination homeopathic formulas, topicals, EFA's, probiotics, etc.

Botanical Alchemy
www.botanicalalchemy.com
800-990-2737
Synergistically blended flower essence formulas.

Dolisos
www.dolisosamerica.com
800-365-4767
Single homeopathic remedies, specialty formulas, throat spray, topicals.

Flower Essence Services
www.fesflowers.com
800-548-0075
Single flower essences, topicals, books, classes.

Green Hope
www.greenhopeessences.com
603-469-3662
Single & combination flower essences.

Natra-Bio
www.natrabio.com
800-232-4005

Specialty homeopathic formulas, vitamins, herbs.

Nelson Bach USA
www.nelsonbach.com
800-319-9151

Single flower essences, topicals, aromatherapy.

Similason
www.healthyrelief.com
800-240-9780
Combination homeopathics – eardrops, nose & throat sprays, eye drops.

Standard Homeopathic/Hyland's
www.hylands.com
800-624-9659
Single homeopathic remedies, specialty formulas, topicals.

Herbs

Clear Products
www.clearproductsinc.com
888-257-2532
Combination herb formulas; Sinus & ear, tinnitis, motion sickness – nausea, migraine & headache.

Eclectic Herbs
www.eclecticherb.com
800-332-4372
Single & combination herb formulas for all ages, ear oil, throat

spray, topicals, prenatal vitamin.

Gaia's Herbs
www.gaiaherbs.com
800-831-7780
Single & combination herbal
formulas for all ages, eardrops,
throat spray, topicals.

Herb Pharm
www.her-pharm.com
800-348-4372
Single & combination herbal
formulas, eardrops, topicals.

Herbs for Kids
www.herbsforkids.com
800-232-4005
Single & specialty herbal formulas,
topicals, eardrops, throat spray,
gum oil.

Highland Laboratories
See nutritional supplements.

IMHOTEP, Inc.
www.imhotepic.com
800-677-8577
Anti-microbial supplements –
ProSeed Grapefruit seed extract
and herbal combination's, ear, nose
& throat, itch spray, feminine rinse,
powder, etc.

Natural Factors
See nutritional supplements.

Nature's Answer
www.naturesanswer.com
800-439-2324
Single & combination herb formulas for all ages, topical homeopath
ic or herbal creams, oral care for
adults.

Nature's Way
www.naturesway.com
800-962-8863
Combination herbal immune
formula, probiotics, EFA's.

New Chapter, Inc.
www.newchapter.info
800-543-7279
Probiotic nutrients, vitamins,
minerals, food & herbal
formulations, topicals.

Renew Life
www.renewlife.com
800-830-4778
Specialty herbal formulas &
nutritional supplements to support
proper digestive health for all ages
over 5 years.

Turtle Island Herbs
www.internatural.com
800-643-4221
Combination herbal formulas,
single plant extracts, throat spray,
itch spray, topicals.

Bath & Skincare Products

Aubrey Organics, Inc
www.aubrey-organics.com
800-282-7394
Hair, skin & body care products for all ages.

Arcona Studio –
Natural Skin Therapy
www.arcona.com
800-657-9991
Original Virtue baby care products, complete line of woman & men skin care & bath products; facial & body treatments; theraputic massage – Hollywood's best-kept secret.

Bella Mama
www.bellamama.com
888-831-4474 or 303-516-0882
Products for pregnancy and new moms; Belly oil, nipple salve, foot salts, sitz bath, etc.

Burt's Bees
www.burtsbees.com
Hair, skin & body care products for all ages.

California Baby
www.californiababy.com
310-277-6430
Hair, skin & body care products, aromatherapy; sunscreen for infants.

Dr. Bronner's Magic Soaps
See non-toxic cleaning products.

Jason's Cosmetics
See oral care section.

Mom's Kiss in a Bottle
www.momskissinabottle.com
877-583-3222
Hair, skin & body care products, aromatherapy.

Nature's Gate
See oral care section.

Trusted Care
www.trustedcare.com
800-458-2811
Hair, skin & body care; unique liquid baby powder.

Well-In-Hand
www.wellinhand.com
888-550-7774
Aromatherapy, medicinal herbal specialty formulas; pregnancy, delivery, yeast, warts, herpes, pain, lice, skin, etc.

Wildflower
www.wildflower.com
888-722-2360/nationwide
323-938-5359/in California
Hair, skin & body care.

V'TAE
www.vtae.com
800-643-3011
Aromatherapy for colds, insomnia, massage and body care

Non-toxic Household Cleaning Products

Dr. Bronner's Magic Soap
www.drbronner.com
760-743-2211

Earth Friendly Products
www.ecos.com
800-335-3267

Ecover
www.ecover.com
800-449-4925

Mountain Green
www.mtngreen.com
866-686-4733

Miscellaneous Healing Tools

CAW Industries
www.dr-willardswater.com
605-343-8100
Willard's water – a catalyst water: can be used topically or internally.

Eco Groovy
www.ecogroovy.com
866-326-4766

Self-heating, re-usable, non-toxic heat packs. (Can be used to help relieve ear pain, cramps, sore muscles, sinus pain, headaches, even to warm a baby's bottle, etc.)

Grampa's Garden, Inc.
www.grampasgarden.com
877-373-4328
Soft comfort aromatherapy line - hot & cold therapy packs (for all ages); essential oils; therapy oil blends, herbal pillows, skin therapy, etc.

Green Sleep
www.greensleep.com
888-413-4442
Cherry pit, hot and cold packs, organic sleep systems, mattresses, cover, pillow.

Heartland Products Inc.
www.licearrest.com
888-772-2345
Lice (rid) foam, shampoo, spray.

Herbal Animals
www.herbal-animals.com
301-469-7800
Aromatherapy herbal animal pillows.

Medic Mates
www.medicmates.com
800-347-4933
Acupressure bands for nausea,

headache, PMS, insomnia; aromatherapy compact carry for sinus, headache, stress and drowsiness.

Natural Relaxer
www.naturalrelaxer.com

301-983-2824
Aromatherapy herbal animal pillows; acupressure bands for nausea, insomnia, headaches and PMS.

Orange Guard, Inc.
www.orangeguard.com
888-659-3217
Non-toxic pest control, ants, roaches, silverfish, etc.

Sea-band International
www.SEA-BAND.com
888-855-2739
Acupressure wristbands for morning sickness (nausea & vomiting), kids sizes for travel sickness, headbands for headaches, and Isocones for insomnia, insect repellent wristband, soothing cool gel pad - feme pad (great for recovery after childbirth); plug-in waterless vaporizer – aromatherapy.

Slumber Sounds
www.slumbersounds.com
866-575-BABY
Kammi teething doll, Ookie – mom's scent doll (first doll), Gripe water, Kiddopotamus – swaddles &

wraps, colic massage oil.

Sneeze-eze
www.sneez-eeze.com
800-247-5731
An inert natural cellulose powder of vegetable origin - nasal spray (for older children.)

Quantum
www.quantumhealth.com
800-448-1448
Lice remover solution & Magic comb, insect repellant, poison ivy/oak relief, sunsceen, cold sore & herpes remedy.

Vapor-eze
www.vaporeze.com
800-343-1240
Aromatherapy – electric waterless vaporizer.

Mail Order Companies

Alternative Pharmacy
www.alternativepharmacy.com
800-578-4104

Apothecarey Pharmacy
www.apothecarey.com
888-399-1777

Capitol Drugs
www.capitoldrugs.com
800-819-9098

Merit Homeopathic –
Knollwood Pharmacy
818-831-1727

Santa Monica Drug
www.smhomeopathic.com
310-395-1131

Product Repertory Resource Guide

Diaper rash
Aloe Life – personal gel
Burt's Bee - cream
California Baby – ointment
Gaia – herbal cream
Eclectic - ointment
New Chapter – Tamanu oil
Weleda - ointment
Well-in-hand – Therapy oil
Wild Flower – ointment

Digestive health & EFA's
(Essential fatty acids)
Aloe Life – aloe, herbs
Barlean's – EFA's
Country Life – probiotic
Health from the Sun – EFA's, fiber
Jarrow Formulas – EFA's, probiotic
Lily of the Desert – aloe, herbs
Naturally Vitamins – Inuflora (prebiotic)
Nature's Way – EFA's, probiotic
Renew Life – herbs, EFA's, probiotic,fiber
Spectrum Essentials – EFA's

Ear
Dolisos – homeopathic combination, syrup
Eclectic Institute – herbal ear drops
Herb Pharm – herbal ear drops
Herbs for Kids – herbal ear drops
Heel/BHI – homeopathic ear drops
Highland Laboratories – herbal liquid

Hyland's – homeopathic combination tablets
Natro-Bio – homeopathic combination, liquid

Eye
Boiron – homeopathic combination drops
Heel/BHI – homeopathic combination drops
Similasan – homeopathic combination drops

Immune
Child Life – herbs, minerals, liquid
Country Life – liquid vitamin C
Eclectic Institute – herbs, liquid & capsules
Enzymatic Therapy – vitamin & herb chewable
Herb Pharm – herbal liquid
Herbs for Kids – herbal liquid
Highland Laboratories – herbal liquid, chewable
Innovative Natural Products – Colloidal formulas
Natural Factors – herbal & vitamin liquids
Nature's Way – herbal liquid
Nutrition Now – herbs, vitamin, mineral chewables
Turtle Island – herbal liquid
Memory/concentration
Enzymatic Therapy
Health from the Sun
Innovative Natural Products
Natrol
Natural Factors
Natures Answer
Renew Life

Nasal applications
Heel/BHI – homeopathic liquid spray
Innovative Natural Products – Aloe & colloidal silver pump
Natro-Bio – homeopathic combination liquid spray

Similason – homeopathic liquid spray
Sneeze-eze – powdered spray
Xlear – liquid spray

Respiratory
Boiron – homeopathic liquid
B & T – homeopathic combination
Dolisos – homeopathic liquid
Gaia Herbs – herbal liquid
Grampa's Herbs – aromatherapy (over 5 years old)
Herb Pharm – herbal liquid
Herbs for Kids – herbal liquid
Highland – rub, herbal liquid, chewable
Nature's Answer – herbal liquid
Turtle Island Herbs – herbal liquid
Ridge Crest – Chinese herbs and combination homeopathic
Vapor-eze – aromatherapy waterless vaporizor

Sinus/Allergy
Capitol Drugs – herbal liquid
Clear Products – herbal capsules
Child Life – herbal liquid
Eclectic – herbal liquid
Herb Pharm – herbal liquid
Herbs for Kids – herbal liquid
Highland Laboratories – herbal chewable
Innovative Natural Products
Nature's Answer – herbal liquid
Turtle Island Herbs – herbal liquid
Vapor-eze – aromatherapy waterless vaporizer

Teething
Boiron USA – homeopathic combination, liquid
Health from the Sun – homeopathic combination oral gel
Herbs for Kids – oral herbal oil
Hyland's – homeopathic combination, tablets & oral gel
Natro-Bio – homeopathic combination, liquid

Heel/BHI – homeopathic oral gel

Throat
Capitol Drugs – herbal, propolis spray
Dolisos – homeopathic
Eclectic – herbal spray
Gaia Herbs – herbal spray
Herbs for Kids – herbal spray
Innovative Natural Products – Colloidal silver spray
ProSeed – herbs & grapefruit seed extract spray
Turtle Island Herbs – herbal combination liquid, spray

Prenatal vitamin
Country Life
Innovative Natural Products
NF Formulas
Rainbow Light
Super Nutrition

Natural alternatives

Clear Products – herbal motion sickness (nausea) capsules
Sea-Band International – Feme pads (cold pack for the vaginal area after childbirth; spatone iron+ supplement)

Lice solutions/insect repellant
Capitol Drugs
Heartland
Orange Guard - bug spray
Quantum
Well-in-hand

Pregnancy, delivery & postpartum
Aloe Life – personal gel (irritated breast or perineum)
Bella Mama – belly oil, nipple salve, sitz bath
Sea-band International - soothing cool pad after childbirth stiches - feme pad

Well-in-hand – New Mama (herb & salts tush soothing bath)

Sunscreen
California Baby – for infants
Jason's Cosmetics
Nature's Gate
Quantum

Recommended Reading List

A Mother's Guide to Raising Healthy Children – Naturally
Sue Frederick
Keats Publishing

Aromatherapy for The Healthy Child
Valerie Ann Worwood
New World Library

Bach Flowers for Children – Raising Emotional Healthy Children Without Drugs
Kathy Arnos
Spirit Dance Publishing

Beyond Antibiotics – Healthier Options for Families
Michael Schmidt, D.C., Lendon Smith, M.D., Keith Sehnert, M.D.
North Atlantic Books

Childhood Ear Infections
Michael Schmidt, D.C.
North Atlantic Books

Don't Drink Your Milk!
Frank A. Oski, M.D.
TEACH Services, Inc.

Dr. Attwood's Low-Fat Prescription for Kids
Charles R. Attwood, M.D.
Penguin Books

Drugs in Pregnancy & Lactaton: A Reference Guide to Fetal & Neonatal Risk - 5th edition
Roger K. Freeman, Sumner J. Yaffe, Gerald G. Briggs, Lippincott, Williams & Wilkins;

Fast Food Nation: The Dark Side Of the All-American Meal
Eric Schlosser
Harper Collins

Feeding Your Child for Lifelong Health
Susan B. Roberts, Ph.D., Melvin B. Heyman, M.D., Lisa Tracy
A Bantam Book

Fluoride: The Aging Factor
John Yiamouyiannis, Ph.D.
Health Action Press

Good Food Today – Great Kids Tomorrow
Jay Gordon, M.D. with Antonia Barnes Boyle
Braun-Brumfield, Inc.
Book or Video

Good Nights: The Happy Parent's Guide to the Family Bed (And a Peaceful Night's Sleep)
Jay Gordon, M.D., Maria Goodavage
Saint Martin's Press
www.drjaygordon.com

Grapefruit Seed Extract, The Authoritative Guide
Allan Sachs, D.C., C.C.N.
LifeRhytum

Healing Gums Naturally
James Harrison, D.D.S., with Constance Clark
Corinthian Health Press

Healthy Parents, Better Babies A Couple's Guide to Natural Preconception Health Care
Francesca Naish,
Janette Roberts
The Crossing Press

Helping The Thumb-Sucking Child
Rosemarie A. Van Norman
Avery Publishing

Kids, Herbs & Health
Linda B. White, M.D., Sunny Mavor
Independent Publishers Group

Homeopathic Family Medicine
(eBook)
Dana Ullman M.P.H.
www.homeopathic.com

Homeopathy A – Z
Dana Ullman M.P.H.
Hay House

How The New Food Labels Can Save Your Life
Peg Jordan, R.N.
Michael Wiese Productions

In Harms Way: Toxic Threats to Child Development
Bernard Weiss, Ph.D., Philip J. Landrigan, M.D.
Greater Boston Physicians for Social Responsibility - Available from NRDC
Natural Resources Defense Council

Is This Your Child? Discovering & Treating Unrecognized Allergies in Children & Adults
Doris Rapp, M.D.
Morrow Publishing

Light, Radiation, & You
John Ott
Devin-Adair Publishers

Listening to your Baby: A New Approach to Parenting Your Newborn
Jay Gordon, M.D.
Perigee Publishing

Medications & Mothers' Milk – 1999-2000
Thomas W. Hale, Ph.D.
Pharmasoft Medical Publications

Milk, Money & Madness: The Culture & Politics of Breastfeeding
Naomi Baumslag, Dia L. Michels, Richard Jolly
Bergin & Garvey

Natural Family Living -The Mothering Magazine Guide to Parenting
Peggy O'Mara
Pocket Books/ Simon & Schuster I

Nature's Pharmacy for Children
Lendon Smith, M.D., Lynne Paige Walker, D. Hom., Ellen Hodgson Brown
Three Rivers Press

No More ADHD
10 steps to help improve your child's attention & behavior without drugs!
Mr. Mary Ann Block
www.blockcenter.com
The Block System
Videos – Learning For-Your-Kids: A program to help develop learning skills - Treat Ear and Respiratory Infections WITHOUT Antibiotics!
800-Dr. Block

Prescription for Nutritional Healing
James F. Balch, M.D., Phyllis A. Balch, C.N.C.
Avery Publishing

Renew Your Life
Brenda Watson, C.T.
Renew Life Press

Ritalin Free Kids
Judyth Reichenberg-Ullman, N.D., Robert Ullman, N.D.
Prima Publishing

Root Canal Cover-Up
George E. Meinig, D.D.S., F.A.C.D.
Bion Publishing

Smart Medicine for A Healthier Child
Janet Zand, L.Ac, O.M.D., Rachel Walton, R.N., Bob Rountree, M.D.
Avery Publishing

Superimmunity for Kids
Leo Galland, M.D., Dian Dincin Buchman, Ph.D.
Dell Publishing

Sweet Dreams – A Pediatrician's Secrets for Baby's Good Night's Sleep
Paul Fleiss, M.D.
Lowell House

The Body Ecology Diet
Donna Gates, Linda Schatz
B.E.D. Publications

The Complete Book of Breastfeeding
Marvin Eiger, M.D.,
Sally Wendkos Olds
Workman Publishing Company

The Complete Book of Dental Remedies
Flora Parsa Stay, D.D.S.
Avery Publishing

The Family Guide to Homeopathy
Andrew Lockie, M.D.
Fireside – Simon & Schuster

The Fragrant Mind
Valerie Ann Worwood
New World Library

The Happiest Baby On the Block
Harvey Karp, M.D.
Random House Publishing
www.thehappiestbaby.com

*The Healing Power of Jerusalem
Artichoke Fiber*
Michael Loes, M.D., M.D.(H.)
Freedom Press

The Natural Pregnancy Book
Aviva Fill Romm
The Crossing Press

The Stevia Cookbook
Ray Sahelian, Donna Gates
Avery Penguin Putnan

*The Stevia Story
A Tale of Incredible Sweetness &
Intrigue*
Linda Bonvie, Bill Bonvie,
Donna Gates
B.E.D. Publications

*The Vaccine Guide: Risks & Benefits
for Children & Adults*
Randall Neustaedter OMD
North Atlantic Books

The Vegetarian Child
Lucy Moll
Perigee – Parenting/Health

Tooth Truth
Frank J. Jerome, D.D.S.
ProMotion Publishing

Toxic Metal Syndrome
Dr. Richard Casdorph, Dr. Morton
Walker
Avery Publishing

Uninformed Consent
Hal Huggins, D.D.S.,
Thomas Levy, M.D.
Hampton Roads Publishing

Why Can't My Child Behave?
Jane Hersey
Pear Tree Press Inc.

Why Raise Ugly Kids?
Hal Huggins, D.D.S.
Crown Publishing

*Wise Woman Herbal for the
Childbearing Year*
Susan S. Weed, Janice Novet
Ash Tree Publications

*Woman's Encyclopedia of
Natural Medicine*
Tori Hudson, N.D.
Keats Publishing

Your Children's Teeth
Theodore Berland,
Alfred Seyler, D.D.S.
Meredith Press

Index

Z

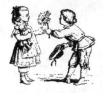